The L.A. Shape Diet

Also by David Heber, M.D., Ph.D.

What Color Is Your Diet?

The L.A. Shape Diet

The 14-Day Total Weight Loss Plan

David Heber, M.D., Ph.D.

with Susan Bowerman, M.S., R.D.

WM

WILLIAM MORROW

An Imprint of HarperCollinsPublishers

NOTE TO READERS

A hardcover edition of this book was published in 2004 by William Morrow, an imprint of HarperCollins Publishers

HarperCollins books may be purchased for educational, business, or sales promotional use. For information please write: Special Markets Department, HarperCollins Publishers Inc., 10 East 53rd Street, New York, NY 10022.

First paperback edition published 2005.

Designed by Joel Avirom

The Library of Congress has cataloged the hardcover edition as follows:

Heber, David.
    The L.A. shape diet : the 14-day total weight loss plan / David Heber with Susan Bowerman—1st ed.
        p. cm.
    ISBN 0-06-073738-7
    1. Reducing diets. 2. Weight loss. I. Title: LA shape diet. II. Bowerman, Susan. III. Title.

RM222.2.H343 2004
613.2'5—dc22

2004041788

ISBN 0-06-075616-0 (pbk.)

14 15 16 WBC/QWF 10 9 8 7 6 5 4 3

*To the source of my inspiration and insight, may this book serve
to work toward the goal that to save one life
is to save the whole world*

Contents

Contents

Introduction

My last book, *What Color Is Your Diet?*, was about how seven simple colors gave clues to the tens of thousands of valuable substances found in fruits and vegetables that, eaten daily, can provide many different health benefits—ranging from the prevention of age-related blindness and mental dysfunction to the prevention of heart disease and many common forms of cancer. This book is about shape—but not the shape of fruits and vegetables.

The L.A. Shape Diet is about the shape of your body and how to change it. Just give me one week to get you started and two weeks to make you feel more lean and fit than ever before. Using the latest scientific knowledge about how your body works and what your diet should be, I'll get you started on a personal journey to a better shape and better health. Personalization is what makes this book different from all the other diet books you have read before—it is about you and your body shape, your diet, and your lifestyle. *The L.A. Shape Diet* is just for you—it's personal!

I developed the philosophy and science behind this book while working with thousands of patients in Los Angeles over the last twenty years. L.A. is a city where shape is important—whether to UCLA students, Hollywood actors, or just ordinary families going to the beach. Everyone wants to look their best, and I will teach you how to get to your best shape in a simple, easy fourteen-day plan complete with menus, recipes, and what I call the Empowering Shake—a drink *you* make that puts you in control of your hunger every day.

Your body shape is related to your body fat, and where this fat is located has a lot to do with how you will lose that fat and what your personal best shape can be. We each have two shapes. The shape we are, and the shape we want to be. Understanding your shape is the first step in getting control of your weight-loss efforts. Lower-body fat is a specialized organ, and its shape is determined by your body's response to female hormones, but only you control how much fat goes to your lower body based on your diet and lifestyle. Studies show that young women often have unrealistic expectations of what their weight should be. They go on one fad diet after another to try to get rid of lower-body fat without success. There is no such thing as spot reducing, but you can personalize your diet and exercise plan to get your personal best body shape.

The fat in the middle of the body is also specialized. This fat stores energy for emergencies by responding to stress hormones, helps you adapt to starvation by controlling hunger, and defends against infections that kill starving people. When you are overweight and there is too much of this fat in your body, it often leads to diabetes and can increase your risks of heart disease and some cancers. Many middle-aged men and women—and their physicians—ignore their modestly expanding waistlines and simply buy larger clothes. A few years ago, I made the same mistake. But the fat surrounding the intestines puts you at risk of serious disease, so you need to do more than simply change the size of your clothes. You will learn how important it is to reduce your waist size as well as your weight so that this fat in the middle of your body works the way it was intended to work. I will show you how thousands of my patients (and I) have managed to lose this fat over the last twenty years.

Your shape gives clues to the body fat, but you need to know more. You need to know how much protein is in your body and how much protein you need in your diet. Most doctors don't measure body protein or consider it in designing your diet. It simply makes sense that the more protein is in your body, the more protein you need to take in to maintain the protein in your muscles and vital organs. Unfortunately, being overweight is often an indication that you have been making poor food choices and not eating enough protein so that your body's protein stores may be run down. Some people avoid eating proteins such as red meat because they think they are fattening, but I will show you how to get enough healthy protein into your diet to combat hunger for the wrong snack foods and to maintain your energy level all day long while you are losing weight. You may be surprised to find that you can diet without hunger for the first time in your life.

Women can have either upper-body or lower-body fat or both, and women need different amounts of protein in the diet based on their personal shape. Those women with upper-body fat and lean thighs have higher male hormone levels and more muscle mass as a rule than women with lower-body fat or an even body fat distribution. As a result, these women tend to have higher protein requirements to maintain their muscle. It's important for these women to know that they have a higher desirable or target weight based on percent body fat than the average woman. When I measure lean body mass and tell these women what their higher target weight is, they are often surprised and usually relieved. I have often heard that I was the first physician to tell a woman that her desirable weight was twenty pounds higher than would be listed on a typical weight-and-height table.

Other women with lower-body fat or average fat distribution can lose muscle mass while they diet. They may look thin, but they still have too much body fat. At the same time, they also have low metabolism, because as you will learn, muscle mass determines the number of calories you burn at rest. Often a combination of exercise, increased protein in the diet, and elimination of hidden fat, sugars, and starches is the first weight-loss approach to work for them.

These are just generalizations. In this book, you will learn how to personalize this information by estimating how much lean and fat *you* have by using some tables in this book, or more precisely through a measurement called "bioelectrical impedance analysis." Beyond the science of this, I know as a doctor that when I give you your personal cholesterol, your personal blood pressure—or, in this case, your personal target weight and your personal best protein and calorie targets—it will impact your behavior much more than some general guidelines suggesting that on average you should eat more of this and less of that.

Seven years ago, I wrote a scientific paper about the importance of estimating body fat and body lean using a simple device called a "bioelectrical impedance meter" to classify the types and degrees of obesity, defined not as excess weight but as excess body fat. I came up with the scientific term "sarcopenic obesity." Sarcopenia means loss of muscle. A woman with sarcopenic obesity is not overweight, so her BMI (Body Mass Index, a weight-to-height ratio) might be only 23, which is within the normal range, but she could easily have excess body fat in the range of 32 to 35 percent. (Normal body fat for women is 22 to 28 percent, and for young, athletic women, it's 15 to 20 percent.) These women may not be getting enough protein on their calorie-reducing diets. As a result, their bodies use up some of the protein in their muscles, their muscle mass goes down, and their metabolism goes down.

The other side of the coin is the large woman who anyone would call overweight. In many cases, these women have much more muscle than other women their height. If they don't get enough protein on a diet, they will be hungry and may just give up trying. In other cases, they succeed in losing the right amount of fat while keeping their lean, but they still weigh more than the tables say they should. Women in commercial weight-loss programs like Weight Watchers have told me they gave up after they couldn't lose weight beyond a certain plateau they had reached. It turned out the plateau was the target weight, and the tables were wrong.

This can happen in men, too. I have seen army officers in the past who were classified as overweight and told to lose weight when they were already at target weight based on fat percentage. I had to write a letter to the commanding officer to straighten things out. Men with more muscle than women often have no difficulty losing weight. They lose weight almost too easily—just cutting their steak in half. This gives them the idea that they can lose weight anytime they want—just as soon as they get around to it. Unfortunately, that is often after their first heart attack or a diagnosis of prostate cancer. *The L.A. Shape Diet* teaches men how much protein to eat along with the latest science on progressive training techniques for building muscle. The fact is that most diets for men never get serious because they don't specify enough protein to keep a large man from being hungry. The Atkins diet was popular with men for just this reason. The average man needs about 150 grams of protein a day, and you have to plan to get that much in a healthy way without all the saturated fat on the Atkins plan. So if you are tired of losing and gaining back the same 20 pounds and never getting the body you want—this book is for you.

To build muscle in people with sarcopenic obesity, and to control appetite in both the sarcopenic and the overmuscular overweight, I have been recommending 1 gram of protein per pound of lean body mass for my patients over the past five years. Take note—this is a key concept. This amount of protein is twice what is recommended now by government advisory groups and equals about 100 grams per day on average for women and 150 grams per day on average for men. Not only will eating more protein maintain your muscle, but there is strong scientific evidence that it will reduce your appetite and make losing weight easier for you. Measurements made in my clinic on 3,500 people using body composition equipment has made it possible for me to set up estimated lean body mass tables to help personalize your weight-loss plan by matching the protein in your diet to the protein in your body. I will also make it simple for you to reach your personal protein goal every day through the use of meal replacements and easy-to-remember food portions of healthy lean meats and fish.

I will design the ideal diet for you starting with the ideal breakfast meal, which I call the Empowering Shake. It provides between 25 and 30 grams of protein, healthy carbohydrates, fiber, vitamins, and minerals, and frankly, it's the best breakfast you can eat. For proof, take a look at the Appendix section, in which I compare the nutrition in the Empowering Shake to the breakfast cereals eaten by millions of Americans every morning.

I recommend powering through the first week by having two protein shakes a day and a healthy meal to get a great start on losing weight and keeping it off for life. On the high-protein shakes that I recommend, not only will you have energy to spare, you'll be able to control your hunger as never before.

The rest of your ideal diet will be built around the colorful fruits and vegetables I wrote about in my last book *What Color Is Your Diet?* The colors of fruits and vegetables are not random. Each of the seven colors that I recommend represents a family of phytochemicals that can affect the function of the cells in your body in different ways. The yellow-green colors found in spinach and avocados represent the lutein family, which is concentrated in one part of the retina in your eye where light is concentrated. Here it protects the eye from age-related macular degeneration, the primary cause of blindness. The red, red/purple, orange, green, white/green, and orange/yellow colors each represent families of compounds called anthocyanins, carotenes, glucosinolates, allyl sulfides, and flavonoids. They are antioxidants that also affect brain function, vision, detoxification, and may help prevent common forms of cancer. These foods also have lots of fiber, enabling you to get close to the 25 grams per day I recommend.

I will also clear up the confusion about carbohydrates by teaching you that not all carbohydrates are bad. You will learn how to use the glycemic index and how to determine the glycemic load and the calories per serving to decide which carbohydrates belong in your ideal diet and which ones to avoid if carbohydrates are a "trigger food" for you. And I go over the other common "trigger foods" that patients tell me tempt them to overeat.

No ideal diet is complete without vitamins and minerals. I will tell you about the most important supplements to take now, and I will tell you about the new breed of vitamins that can provide the phytochemicals normally found in fruits and vegetables in concentrated form in tablets and gelatin capsules. These are important additions to the diet, because fruits and vegetables don't always deliver the optimum amounts of these important substances, and it may be hard to always eat the seven servings that I recommend.

Losing weight is like a road trip. You need to know where you are going and how you are going to get there. Beyond nutrition, you will learn about behavior, exercise, building muscle, spirituality and inner vision, and about herbal supplements that may help you get over some roadblocks along the way. However, it is important to remember that there are no magic pills that will enable you to eat whatever you want and still lose weight. On the other hand, this is not rocket science. I believe that I can teach you how to lose weight along with the thousands of patients I have seen in the last twenty years.

I am a physician and a professor of medicine and public health. The word "doctor" comes from the Latin root for teacher, so I am a teacher twice over. I am also a doctor twice over, being both an M.D. (medical doctor) and a Ph.D. (doctor of philosophy) in physiology. I see patients during the week and on some Saturdays, and I supervise a large research group of seven professors, seven fellows, and a thirty-five-member staff at the UCLA Center for Human Nutrition, which I established in 1996. I also direct one of the largest and most successful weight management programs in the country, the Risk Factor Obesity Clinic at UCLA. This program has treated thousands of patients and touched countless lives. One of my greatest rewards is changing the lives of my patients by helping them lose weight and keep it off. I see all kinds of patients, including captains of industry, entertainers, dedicated grade school teachers, nurses, other doctors, architects, psychologists, and psychiatrists. The program in this book is based both on my research and my practice with patients every day.

Recently, I became the chairman of the Scientific and Medical Advisory Board of Herbalife International, which has over one million distributors in fifty-nine countries. In addition to many of my colleagues in the field of obesity treatment, Dr. Louis Ignarro, the first Nobel prizewinner at the UCLA School of Medicine, has joined me on this advisory board. Herbalife has adopted many of the principles in this book, including the personalization of nutritional advice based on body composition, and I am extremely grateful to them for providing me with the opportunity to get my message out to tens of millions of people.

If you pick up this book and you benefit from it, please tell a friend. Obesity is a worldwide problem that will require a worldwide solution. Please be a part of this solution.

David Heber, M.D., Ph.D.
Los Angeles, California
November 2003

Changing Your Shape

You know when you feel "in shape"—your waist is more defined and your muscles are more fit. In fact, muscle weighs more than fat per unit volume, so it is possible to lose fat and not weight if you're following a diet program that involves exercising.

For some people, losing weight is not the most urgent problem, although it is certainly a part of it. These people mainly need to remodel their bodies by gaining muscle and losing fat. Let me speak from personal experience. If you had met me three years ago, you wouldn't have thought I was obese. At that time I was 5 feet 11 inches tall and about 192 pounds, with a waist size of 36 inches. I knew I wasn't in my best shape. No one else knew I was fat. I was getting away with it, but I had extra fat on my chest and around my neck and face. I could think back to college, when I went from a pudgy 192 pounds down to 172 pounds by eating cottage cheese and burger patties. I was eighteen then, and now I was fifty-four, so that fat came on in different places, and it was going to be harder to lose.

I was getting away with my extra fat around the middle until I took a trip to Denver, Colorado, for a meeting held in The Brown Palace Hotel. This hotel has an older wing in which, for some reason, you have to step up from the room to get into a cramped bathroom. Well, I saw the step on the way in, but on the way out—whoops! I twisted my right knee and hit the wall about a foot away from the bathroom door. My knee bothered me the rest of the night and for weeks afterward. I tried bed rest and pain relievers and in the process gained 24 pounds. My waist grew to 38 inches, and I had to buy some new pants.

Two months later, after a very long flight to Holland, I worked out on a bicycle in a hotel gym and felt a sudden rip of pain in the same knee I had injured in Denver. It was so bad that on the flight back I called my orthopedist from the plane to make an appointment the day I arrived home. He recommended surgery right away, but I had a trip to Japan coming up and wanted to make one more attempt to rehabilitate my knee. So I went on the weight-loss program you will read about in this book, with high-protein shakes, daily exercise, and fruits and vegetables. My body fat has decreased from 21 percent to 17 percent, and my waist has gone from a 38 to a 34. But I lost just 24 pounds, going from 204 to 180. What's most important is that my shape has changed. I have lost weight around the middle and gained muscle weight in my arms. I feel better, and I avoided knee surgery.

I didn't tell this story to brag about my weight loss, because I didn't lose that much weight. What is most important is where I lost the weight. I lost fat in my abdomen and gained muscle weight in my arms. My health improved out of proportion to my weight loss.

As someone who teaches both doctors and the public about obesity, I believe weight loss has been overemphasized and body fat underemphasized. You have probably read about the Body Mass Index, which is a weight-to-height ratio. If your BMI is greater than 25 you are considered overweight in the United States, and if it is greater than 30, you are obese. (You can determine your BMI using the table on page 47). This ratio has been a powerful way for scientists to document the obesity epidemic in this country and its effects on health and disease. However, when it comes to you as an individual, it can be misleading.

A football player can be considered overweight on the BMI scale and not overfat if the extra weight being carried is muscle, not fat. A thin woman can have a normal BMI and be overfat. In fact, in a study of young women in our clinics at UCLA, I found a lot of women with a BMI of 23 (in the healthy range) who had a percent body fat that was too high at 32 percent. So shapes can be deceiving, but for your personal shape there is a best weight based on the lean-to-fat ratio.

We can categorize shapes into two types: the shape you can change and the shape you can't change. Of course, it is important to know the difference and change the shape you can change while adjusting your wardrobe and your attitudes to live with the shape you can't change. I have great sympathy for overweight patients, but I can't ask you to adjust to an unhealthy level of body fat to protect these overweight patients from ridicule. In other words, I can't say fat is beautiful. I can say let us appreciate all the shapes of different people at a healthy body weight with healthy amounts of body fat.

Tools for Changing Your Shape

Most diet books have some "big" secret, such as cutting almost all carbohydrates or fats out of the diet. The promise is that if you do this one simple thing, you will lose weight and be able to keep eating almost the same way you are now without having to give up the foods you love. But if you don't like your shape, one simple trick won't change things. There are probably several things wrong with your diet and lifestyle at the very same time.

What you need is a personalized plan. One size doesn't fit every overweight person; people come in different shapes and sizes. And until you can describe your shape accurately, you're not ready to make your personal plan for losing weight and keeping it off. So, what is your shape? Are you an apple or a pear? Are you big or small? Are you fat or lean?

Finding Your Shape Silhouette

Look at the figures below and pick a shape closest to your own.

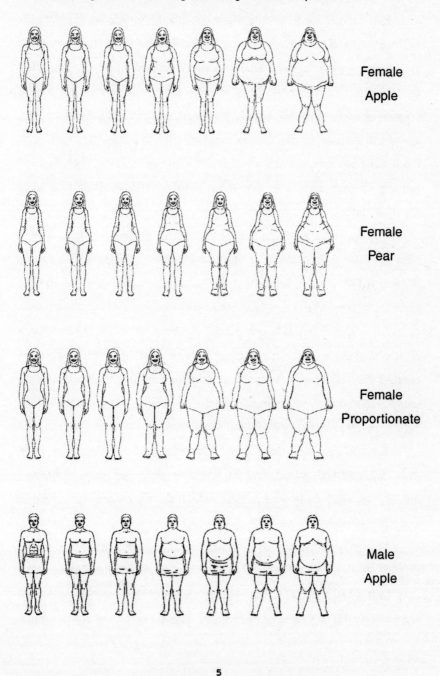

Female
Apple

Female
Pear

Female
Proportionate

Male
Apple

Why Shape Makes a Difference

Apple-shaped people have upper body fat. The fat cells in the upper body, including the face, neck, breasts, and waist, behave differently than fat cells in the thighs and hips. The upper-body fat cells are there to help both men and women withstand periods of starvation—which happened quite often in ancient times. The lower-body fat cells help women store fat during pregnancy so that they will have enough stored calories to provide an average of 500 calories per day as breast milk in order to nurse a newborn baby. Until fairly recently, women spent much more of their lives bearing and nursing children, so this fat gave them a real advantage, along with fat in the upper body.

The upper-body fat that is held around the intestines, which is seen on the outside as an increase in waist size (and on the inside with a special X-ray called a CT scan), is even more specialized. This fat tissue sends fatty acids to the liver and causes changes in your insulin levels that affect how much fat you store versus how much fat you burn. When there is too much of this fat in the body, it can also cause inflammation in various tissues, including the heart. Losing weight around your neck, face, chest, and waist usually goes along with losing fat on the inside. So, as you begin to look better, you also improve your health tremendously.

But you can't lose these special fat cells just by dieting, which can cause a loss of both muscle and fat. You have to change your lifestyle and exercise to build some lean muscle, which then remodels your percent body fat and body lean.

Pear-shaped women have lower-body fat, found on the hips and thighs. Men may be thinner or heavier around the hips and thighs, but they don't get this type of fat unless they are very old or have low male hormone levels due to illness or medication. This fat is not medically dangerous, but ever since Twiggy landed on our shores from England it has made women miserable. These lower-body fat cells are resistant to exercise and diet; if women have a low metabolism, they won't be able to lose weight even when they cut calories. You have to take special steps to get enough protein to control your cravings and maintain or build muscle to get the shape you want.

So, losing weight is harder if you have lower-body fat rather than upper-body fat, but the medical benefits of losing your upper-body fat are greater. Luckily, as you lose upper-body fat, you will lose some lower-body fat as well.

I'll teach you how to get to your personal target weight and body fat level, and then you will be able to judge how you feel about your new shape. Knowing that you have the right shape for *you* may finally allow you to get off the dieting roller coaster and get on with the rest of your life.

Six Steps to Success

My purpose in this book is to teach you how to change your shape while motivating and inspiring you to change. This means that you must be a part of the solution. Together we will develop a schedule for changing your shape. I will provide you with the six steps, but you need to take them.

First, I will empower you to get through that first week of change with a simple meal replacement plan that I have used with thousands of patients. Twice a day, you'll have two very high-protein shakes, made with fruit in a blender. I call this the Empowering Shake, because it tastes better than anything you'll find in a can and it will provide the amount of protein matched to your body's needs. It will satisfy your hunger and help you gain control of your food choices during the day. This jump-start week will give you the kind of results that inspire you to go on. You'll lose weight and water and will feel better right away. I know this system works, but the choice is up to you. If you don't want this quick start you can go on to a two-week plan in which you drink one shake per day, with a more gradual loss of weight. If you can drink the two shakes daily and keep it up until you reach your goal, you should try to do so, because your results will be faster.

Second, I'll personalize your program by teaching you snack defenses for particular Trigger Foods. You'll also learn your appropriate target weight so that you will not only end up at the right body weight but the right ratio of fat to lean. You'll personalize your protein intake to enable you to control your hunger and cravings for the wrong foods. Armed with all this information, you'll build your personal diet plan.

Third, you'll learn shopping, dining out, traveling, and holiday eating solutions. You'll learn to reorganize your pantry in order to change your home food environment. I'll also provide you with simple and easy recipes, and a few fancier and yet still healthy recipes for special occasions.

Fourth, I'll teach you about relapse prevention and the underlying causes of poor behavior patterns that can sabotage your efforts to lose weight. You'll learn the skills of self-talk and how to keep an effective emotional diary. You'll learn how to change patterns of behavior by recognizing them for what they are. Finally, you'll learn how to avoid the trap of self-destructive behavior as I teach you how not to rain on your own parade.

Fifth, I'll inspire you to increase your confidence in your ultimate success. I'll share many success stories with you drawn from my own experience that will enable you to visualize your personal success. And I'll suggest ways that you can effectively reward yourself to maintain your momentum.

Sixth, you'll indulge in what I call "the only healthy addiction" and bring the habit of exercise into your life. I'll teach you how to make a space in your home and in your life for the exercise you need to correct a sedentary lifestyle. Left unchecked, being sedentary is a disease that dissolves your muscles and bones slowly and imperceptibly over decades, causing you to age prematurely.

So there it is. Changing your shape in six easy steps. There is information in the Appendix on the proper vitamins, minerals, and some of the herbal supplements that have been studied for weight loss. I will provide you with my best evaluation of these supplements and recommend that you only use them together with a diet and lifestyle program to increase the rate of your weight loss. I am against the idea of magic pills or magic herbs. I have included the science behind much of what is written in this book in the appendix as separate sections of the science behind shape and body fat, meal replacements, bioelectrical impedance analysis, protein, good and bad fats, cereals versus shakes, exercise and building muscle, and vitamins and minerals. These sections are designed for those who want to know more about the science behind the six easy steps to changing your shape.

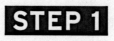

Power Through the First Week

The beginning of any great adventure is momentous. Before you start to change your shape, you need to be ready to make a change in your life. Think carefully and be sure that you are ready to make a change now. If you are, I am ready with the information and tools you will need to make a great start. For this first week, we are going to skip any fancy calculations, and I am going to give you a simple program to follow. I am doing this because it will make it easier for you to start the program. (If you are one of those people who likes to do things precisely, then you can skip ahead to calculate your exact protein needs for this first week.)

In this chapter, I'll empower you by teaching you how to use protein to get control of your eating every day. Then I will give you a choice to make. You can jump-start your plan to lose weight by using meal replacements, which have been scientifically proven to make calorie control easier, or you can simply try to eat foods in controlled portions to try to accomplish the same thing.

I must warn you that this second approach may sound more appealing, but it is difficult just to decrease the amounts of your favorite foods and still get adequate protein, vitamins, and minerals on a diet. In research studies, trying simply to eat less of your favorite foods works the least well of all approaches to weight loss.

How Weight Loss Works

If you eat the same number of calories as you burn, your weight remains the same:

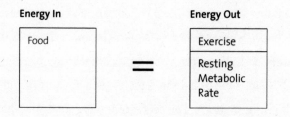

If you eat fewer calories than you burn, you lose weight, and for every 500 calories less you eat per day, you will lose about 1 pound of weight per week:

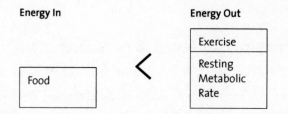

The amount of food you eat is less than the calories you burn, but the energy has to come from somewhere. Your body takes it from your stored calories of fat, and whenever you take in 500 calories less per day than your body needs, it burns one pound of fat in a week. So, if you eat 250 calories less than you burn each day, you will lose ½ pound per week, and if you eat 1,000 calories less per day, you will lose 2 pounds per week and so forth. The key to healthy weight loss is to make sure the reduced calories you eat provide the nutrition you need. And the key to effective weight management is to make sure that the foods delivering those reduced calories are enjoyable and satisfying.

The Secret of High-Protein Brain Signals

High-protein foods send signals to the brain that keep you from being hungry for hours—stronger signals than either carbohydrate or fat gives. As the protein in your food is digested in your intestines, it is broken down to individual building blocks of protein called "amino acids." Some of these can enter the brain, where they can affect the balance of signals that monitor how hungry or full you are. Our typical breakfasts of refined cereal grains often have too little protein in them to send the kind of signal of fullness that will last until lunch. The secret of the Empowering Shake is that it will keep you feeling full—*if* you put enough protein into it. As you will see, this is more protein than you think, and very likely more than you are eating now.

The Protein You Need Every Day

If you eat too little protein, you can damage your heart and muscles seriously. This was a problem with some of the starvation diets of the 1970s. The next generation of meal replacements provided enough protein to avoid these problems. When used as recommended, the meal replacement plans of the 1980s used two shakes and a regular meal, and provided about 50 to 70 grams of protein in one day. But a lot of people complained of hunger within a few hours of drinking these lower-protein shakes. Then, in the 1990s, the tide turned and the market favored low-carbohydrate diets with high-fat and high-protein shakes. These were much more filling, but as you will see later the low-carbohydrate part of these diets is not healthy, and the truth is that you don't need all that fat to feel full.

The Empowering Shake is satisfying because it has enough protein to match your body's needs. It makes sense that a 250-pound man is going to need more protein than a 120-pound woman to feel satisfied. I'll show you how to make an Empowering Shake with your personalized protein prescription, but first I want to give you an idea of some typical plans for protein consumption.

For a typical woman, I recommend about 100 grams of protein per day. That would be 25 to 30 grams at breakfast and lunch as a shake, a 25-gram protein snack in the late afternoon, and at dinner a salad made with up to 4 cups of lettuce with wine or rice vinegar, 5 ounces of chicken or fish with 3 cups of steamed vegetables, and a fruit for dessert. For a typical man, I recommend 150 grams of protein per day: 30 to 40 grams each for breakfast and lunch, 20 to 30 grams in the afternoon snack, and 50 to 75 grams at dinner.

Personalizing Your Protein Intake

How do you personalize all these different protein levels when you make your shake? I do this by combining a soy-protein shake with soy milk or regular nonfat milk. The meal replacement shake mix I use has about 10 grams of protein per serving, and the soy milk or nonfat milk adds another 10 grams of protein. I then add a protein powder supplement with another 5 grams for a 25-gram protein breakfast or another 10 grams (as two scoops) for a 30-gram breakfast.

In this first week, I want to keep things simple. Start with the previous average recommendations. If you find that you're hungry a few hours after consuming a shake with 25 grams of protein, for your next shake, add another one or two scoops of protein powder supplement with about 5 grams of protein per scoop. I add two scoops to my shake, making the total protein content over 35 grams. Two 35-gram shakes in a day will give you

70 grams of protein. Now, at dinner, if you eat a 6-ounce portion of chicken, lean meats, turkey, fish, or soy meat substitute, you add another 50 grams, for a total of 120 grams for the day. This is above the recommended protein for the average woman (100 grams) and below that for the average man (150 grams), but you can adjust as necessary later in the week or in the second week by estimating your protein needs (see page 48).

Anyone who is dieting should get a minimum of 50 grams of protein per day to be safe. This is the safe but hunger-prone meal replacement plan of the 1980s. You should never take in less than this amount. You could get this 50 grams of protein from two 12-gram meal replacement shakes, without added pure protein powder, and a dinner with one 3-ounce meat serving. There are many meal replacement shakes on the market that meet this criterion, but I believe that on this amount of protein you will feel hungry and be tempted to go off the plan. Meal replacements can deliver this when used properly, and there are a number of studies, including some from my laboratories at UCLA, that show how well meal replacements work by simplifying calorie control.

Jump-Start Your Plan

Over the last twenty years, I have been involved in research that has proven the safety and effectiveness of meal replacement shakes to jump-start a lifelong diet plan. The key to losing weight is creating a difference between what you eat every day and what you need to burn to maintain your body at rest and during exercise. If you can just reduce your calorie intake by 500 calories per day below what you burn, you will lose 1 pound per week. Unless you burn more than 3,000 calories per day, that is about all you can expect to lose once you get past the first week—1 to 2 pounds per week. If you think about it, that is 50 to 100 pounds in one year. To lose any more quickly than 2 pounds per week is unhealthy and you simply can't expect to lose 20 pounds in a week or two.

The first week you will likely lose 5 pounds or more, due to the loss of excess salt and water from your body. Insulin, which is known as the feeding hormone, causes your body to hold on to extra salt and water when you are heavy. In that first week, as your insulin levels fall in response to the decrease in the number of calories you consume, you lose over a quart of water more than you take in. Since each quart weighs about 2 pounds, you can estimate that half of the first 5 pounds lost that first week comes from water and salt losses. However, you will definitely feel lighter and have the satisfaction of seeing the number on the scale go lower. If you go off your plan and start eating more calories, this weight will come back quickly again as salt and water. Just get right back to your plan. No one gains 3 to 5 pounds of fat in a day, and this salt and water will come off as easily as it went on you in just a few days.

To achieve this savings of 500 calories per day in order to lose a pound a week, you need a way to control calories. But it is almost impossible to count calories, because of the hidden fat, sugar, and starch in processed food and restaurant food as well as the larger portion sizes that are served today. Food labels are confusing, and it is difficult to know how to combine individual foods into a healthy diet based on the information you find on a food label. High-protein shakes will not only give you energy and help you control your hunger, but you will know with certainty how many calories you are taking in so that you can organize your ideal personal diet plan.

The Empowering Shake

Making your own high-protein shake puts you in control of your protein intake, your hunger level, and ultimately your weight loss. The Empowering Shake is the twenty-first-century meal replacement, with fruit, soy protein, and calcium all in one delicious package.

I recommend using a meal replacement powder made with about 10 grams of soy protein isolate containing specified amounts of soy isoflavones, healthy carbohydrate, fiber, vitamins and minerals, and a protein booster powder that provides 5 grams of protein per tablespoon. This protein booster allows you to individualize the amounts of protein in your Empowering Shake. For example, I use 2 tablespoons of the protein booster to increase the total protein in my Empowering Shake to a total of 29 grams.

Follow these simple steps to set up a shake preparation area in your kitchen.

Get a good blender and keep it clean. Blenders are relatively inexpensive; they run anywhere from $30 to $50 on sale. Buy one you like, because you'll be using it every morning.

Keep your protein powder and/or meal replacement powders in a cabinet near the blender and have your measuring spoon or scoop handy. Know how much of each powdered protein ingredient you plan to add to your blender to reach your protein goal.

Have nonfat milk or plain soy milk available. I like to buy soy milk in the small boxes (called tetra-pak containers) that don't need to be refrigerated until you open them.

Buy fresh or frozen fruits to add to your shake. I usually add a cup of frozen blueberries, but you can use banana, mango, pineapple, or strawberries.

Now that you are ready, here's the exact order in which you'll mix the ingredients to make this delicious shake:

1   Add 8 ounces of soy milk or nonfat dairy milk to the blender (for 10 grams of protein to start).

2   Add the desired amount of meal replacement powder.

3   Add the amount of protein powder that in combination with your meal replacement powder will enable you to reach your daily protein target (see page 15, "Personalizing Your Protein Intake").

4   Add 1 cup of fresh fruit (blueberries, strawberries, or banana) and 2 to 4 ice cubes, or 1 cup of frozen fruit (ice is optional).

5   Some blenders come with a smoothie drink program. If you don't have this, then start slow to get everything mixed, and then speed up in pulses to be sure that the frozen fruit or ice is chopped up until you get the consistency of a smoothie. If you use fresh fruit, you will get a thinner consistency. By adding ice cubes or frozen fruits you can get to the consistency of an ice cream or a milk shake depending on how much ice you add.

6   Drink or eat your shake with a spoon over ten to fifteen minutes. By eating slowly you allow your system to digest your shake, and you practice eating more slowly for other meals throughout the day.

7   Rinse out your glass and the blender with lots of warm water right away, and you won't have problems keeping your blender clean.

There is no better way to make a shake. Ready-to-drink shakes in cans or packs are limited by their ability to dissolve protein, which settles at the bottom if there is not enough fat to suspend it. If you look at most high-protein shakes, you will see lots of fat—sometimes 8 or 9 grams. Ready-to-drink high protein shakes can be a convenient mid-day or late afternoon snack with a fruit or vegetable when you are on the go. Just remember to look at the label carefully and try to get a shake that has 5 grams or less of fat and 10 to 15 grams of protein.

Jump-Start Diet for Week 1, or Shake-Shake-Meal!

You have the power to change yourself. You may not be able to change your job, the traffic, the weather, or your relatives, but you can change yourself. All it takes is a plan. Give me just one week to start you on the road to a life-time weight management plan. Pick a day to start, buy your supplies, and get going.

I recommend that you use two meal replacements a day to power through the first week, but you can use one shake for breakfast and eat a portion-controlled lunch for a slower weight loss if this seems like too much for you right now. Each meal replacement Empowering Shake is customized to your personal protein needs by adding two tablespoons of pure protein powder to your meal replacement powder and nonfat dairy or soy milk to reach your daily protein target (see pages 48–49).

As you plan your third meal (or in some cases both lunch and dinner), you should keep it simple. Basically, this meal will consist of 3 to 6 ounces of chicken, fish, or turkey, 2 cups of steamed vegetables, 4 cups of salad with rice or wine vinegar, and a fruit for dessert. In Step 2, you will get more ideas on how to put together delicious meals.

Your First Seven Days

You can see the plan for the first seven days of shake-shake-meal below. There are lots of different flavor suggestions for the shakes, but you don't need to try them all. If you find one you like, you can use that flavor all week—but do know that people often lose ambition to follow dietary programs when they start to feel bored, so throw in some variety to keep yourself interested.

You can use spices on your vegetables and fruits. Making a baked apple with cinnamon can make it taste like a slice of apple pie and it has only about 100 calories compared to a slice of apple pie which has just over 400 calories. Recent research suggests that cinnamon may be a good idea when you are losing weight. For vegetables, seasoning is a great way to make your "greens" tastier. You can also use salsa or tomato sauce, and the good news is that most spices are free of significant calories, plus you can use salt and pepper or even chili powder as much as you want. Chili has also been studied for its ability to be an aid to weight loss.

Day One:

Breakfast:	*Pumpkin Banana Shake
Lunch:	*Chocolate Raspberry Shake
Snack:	1 ounce roasted soy nuts—about ⅛ cup
Dinner:	*Quick Chicken Soup
	Tossed Green Salad with *L.A. Shape Dressing

Day Two:

Breakfast:	*Strawberry Kiwi Shake
Lunch:	*Chai Tea Latte Shake
Snack:	½ protein bar (to supply about 125 calories and 10 grams protein)

Dinner:	*Baja Seafood Cocktail
	Tossed Green Salad with *L.A. Shape Dressing

Day Three:

Breakfast:	*Banana Walnut Shake
Lunch:	*Pineapple-Orange-Coconut Shake
Snack:	½ cup nonfat cottage cheese + ½ cup fresh fruit
Dinner:	Grilled chicken, turkey, shrimp, or fish and vegetable
	kabobs with 2 tablespoons barbecue sauce
	Chopped vegetable salad

Day Four:

Breakfast:	*Very Berry Shake
Lunch:	*Orange Mango Shake
Snack:	2 ounces roasted turkey breast + ½ cup baby carrots
Dinner:	*Oven-"Fried" Fish
	Steamed broccoli and carrots
	Tossed salad with *L.A. Shape dressing

Day Five:

Breakfast:	*Chocolate Strawberry Shake
Lunch:	*Orange Julius Shake
Snack:	¾ cup plain yogurt + ½ cup fruit
	or one 8-ounce carton fat-free, sugar-free yogurt
Dinner:	*Asian Lettuce Cups
	Steamed mixed vegetables

Day Six:

Breakfast:	*Pina Colada Shake
Lunch:	*Peach Almond Shake
Snack:	½ high-protein bar and an apple

Dinner:	*Juicy Roast Turkey Breast
	Steamed butternut squash
	*Healthy Cabbage Slaw

Day Seven:

Breakfast:	*Café Mocha Shake
Lunch:	*Blueberry-Cranberry Shake
Snack:	1 individual 3-ounce can tuna + 1 cup tomato juice or mixed vegetable juice
Dinner:	*Spicy Jamaican Chicken
	Steamed carrots with lemon and dill
	Sliced tomatoes with basil

*Recipes begin on page 102.

Drinking Water Is Important

One of the most important things you can do when dieting is to drink enough water. You should normally drink three to four 8-ounce glasses of water per day. You will find that your afternoon fatigue is often due to dehydration and will improve by paying attention to your water intake. If you are exercising or the weather is hot, drinking water is even more important, as you lose it through sweating. But don't overdo it. If you drink two quarts (eight 8-ounce glasses) of water per day, you can literally become water-logged and will note swelling in your hands and feet. Some diets recommend this amount each day as a trick to keep your stomach filled. This is a mistake, and in some people it can lead to problems. This is a rare problem, but it does happen. I see this sometimes in patients who drink water from quart-size bottles while they speak to me. This is a nervous habit, but of course it has a medical name: psychogenic polydipsia.

Drinking tea in the afternoon, especially green tea, can be a great energy booster. Studies have shown that green tea can stimulate metabolism by about 80 calories a day when you drink four to six teacups per day or take a supplement containing green tea (see Step 7). The caffeine in both coffee and tea acts on your kidneys to increase urine flow. So tea and coffee don't count toward your water intake because they cause your kidneys to excrete more water than they contain.

Getting Your Vitamins and Minerals on a Diet

Many meal replacement powders contain some vitamins and minerals, usually at a fraction of the Recommended Dietary Allowance, or RDA, you need each day. Colorful fruits and vegetables also provide many vitamins and minerals, but you should be sure to take a multivitamin/multimineral supplement whenever you are eating a less-than-varied diet. It is a good idea in general and will guarantee adequate folic acid intake. Not only is folic acid included in most supplements at 400 micrograms per day, but folic acid is better absorbed from vitamins than from food sources. Daily doses of multivitamins also provide adequate amounts of many other key vitamins and minerals. Women and men under age fifty should consume 1,000 milligrams of calcium daily from the diet and supplements, while women over fifty should consume a total of 1,500 milligrams of calcium. Look at the calcium content in your foods and soy shake, and be sure to add them all together in figuring out how much calcium is in your diet. You will likely not need to supplement calcium, but it depends on how many shakes per day you are using, and how much calcium they contain. If you need a calcium supplement, take one with vitamin D in it.

Troubleshooting Common Complaints

"I FEEL WEAK AND TIRED."

In some people, overeating stimulates their nervous system much like a strong cup of coffee, causing sweating and making their pulse more rapid. After a while, this just seems normal to some overweight people. As soon as these people begin to diet, their nervous system settles down to normal and they complain of not feeling as alert or energetic. When I encounter this problem, I simply tell my patients that they now have normal energy levels and need proper rest and sleep when they get tired. After a period of adjustment, they will feel more energetic again.

You may also feel weak and tired if you don't consume your meal replacement shakes at regular times. Are you accidentally forgetting to eat lunch, or are you skipping meals in an attempt to lose weight faster? This is a mistake, since you will always eat more trying to recover from fatigue than you save by skipping a meal or shake.

"I'M NOT REGULAR."

Whenever you change your diet, your digestive function can change. You may not be having regular bowel movements, or you may be producing extra gas. You'll feel better if you consume 25 grams of fiber a day. The easiest way to get this fiber is to eat fruits and vegetables. If you can't get the 25 grams from fruits and vegetables then there are fiber supplements available with a mixture of soluble and insoluble fibers that can help with regularity. Some of the newest fibers can be mixed into beverages without giving any gritty taste and can provide 5 grams of fiber per tablespoon.

"I'M HUNGRY ALL THE TIME."

There are usually two different causes for true hunger. First, you may be forgetting meals or letting too much time elapse between meals. Put yourself on a regular schedule—such as 7 A.M., 11 A.M., 4 P.M., and 7 P.M.—for your meal replacement, snacks, and meals. The second common cause is inadequate protein intake. Check your meal replacement and make sure that it has as much protein per serving as you're counting on. Also, be sure you are physically hungry and not just craving your favorite foods. I'll discuss Trigger Foods and ways to conquer them in Step 4.

"I HAVE A HEADACHE."

Constipation, stress, and missed meals are the most common causes of headaches when you're in your first week of dieting. If you're constipated, try one of the preceding suggestions. Stress headaches begin with muscle spasms in the shoulders and spread to the scalp, where the spasms cut off the blood flow to the scalp, causing a headache. Check out some of the remedies for stress in Step 5. And as I've mentioned, it's very important not to miss meals.

Some people also get headaches from caffeine withdrawal, but as far as I'm concerned, there's no need for you to cut out caffeine. Coffee in the usual amounts of 1 or 2 cups per day is safe during dieting, and may actually help with your weight loss.

"I FEEL COLD."

Your body temperature actually increases when you overeat. Many of my patients come in sweating before starting a diet, and then one week later they feel terrific. On the other hand, dieting may make you more sensitive to temperature changes. Exercising, drinking warm tea and coffee, and dressing warmly in cold weather are all good solutions to this common complaint. While unusual, feeling cold can be a symptom of low thyroid gland function. So, if a cold feeling persists, talk to your doctor.

You won't necessarily have any of the complaints I have listed. Don't fall for the old medical student problem of reading about a disease and getting it. Most of my patients have none of these complaints and tell me that this weight-loss plan does not involve a lot of hunger and suffering, as some others have. However, if you feel you need a dietary supplement to help control your appetite, stimulate your metabolism, or help your fat cells release fat more effectively, read Step 6 for some ideas.

Now that you have made a great start in the first seven days, Step 2 will take you into the next seven days with menus and recipes that you can use over the long term to lose weight and keep it off.

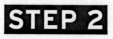

Personalizing Your Program

Most diets give you something while taking something else away. This is the same tactic you use to get a dangerous toy away from a dog. As you take the toy away, you entice the dog with a tasty treat.

The low-fat diets, such as the Pritikin, take away the fat and give you lots of grains, beans, fruits, and vegetables, with limited protein. The lack of protein leads some people to get hungry and overeat starchy foods. It is real news to some people that a cup of beans, rice, or potato contains 250 calories. A simple bowl of lentil soup can contain 500 calories. Limiting fat while allowing starchy and refined carbohydrates is very healthy as long as you burn off the extra calories. As a weight-loss plan, it doesn't work well.

At the other end of the spectrum, the Atkins diet takes away the carbohydrates and gives you back the fatty red meats and cheeses that were restricted on the low-fat diets. The Atkins diet in its original version was obsessed with cutting out all carbohydrates including the healthy ones found in fruits, vegetables, and real whole grains. At the same time, Atkins allows you to eat unlimited amounts of bacon and other tasty-sounding treats. Much like a kid in a candy store, eating all the bacon and cheese you want sounds great—for a while. But my experience is that many people ultimately end up craving carbohydrates again. In the end, you haven't changed your taste buds, and you gain back the weight you lost. Toward the end of his life, Dr. Atkins did broaden the dietary choices to include some vegetables, and most people on what they think is the Atkins diet are really on a modified Atkins diet, where they eat some vegetables and fruits.

You can learn from these two opposing views. Scientific studies summarized in the Appendix show that protein is more satisfying than fat over the short term. I believe it is the protein in the Atkins diet that accounts for its success. Atkins coupled a bit of truth (protein helps control hunger) with a license to eat all the "forbidden" foods, including high-fat foods. The problem is that fat calories are hidden in many foods and can sneak into you without filling you up. So it's important to cut fat to a reasonable level, at which you use just enough to maintain good flavor and maintain the heat in the foods you prepare. This amounts to about 20 percent of calories from fat.

The Atkins formula was trotted out twice—first in the 1960s and then in the late 1990s, after the Zone diet gave you permission to eat 30 percent fat in the mid-1990s. The Zone diet was published in 1995. The Atkins diet advises a remarkable 59 percent of calories from fat, along with 36 percent from protein. The diet leaves almost no room for healthy carbohydrates, at 5 percent of total calories. Healthy carbohydrates like colorful fruits and vegetables are rich in fiber, vitamins, minerals, and phytonutrients, and should not be eliminated solely because they are carbs. Nothing is new under the sun, and the original high-fat, high-protein diet was suggested more than 200 years ago by an undertaker to an overweight English king. Those who make money from the sales of high-fat foods were thrilled with the Atkins diet, and a columnist for the *New York Times* accused the scientific community of lying to the public for a decade about the fact that high-fat diets lead to weight gain. We didn't lie—fat will still make you fat. It is just more complicated, and scientists have begun to emphasize the impact of the amount of protein in the diet. We have also begun to consider the effects on blood sugar levels and insulin levels of sugar and starch in comparison to those of real whole grains (otherwise known as glycemic index and glycemic load), which I'll discuss shortly.

A recent entrant in the popular diet derby is "Dr. Phil" McGraw, a Ph.D. clinical psychologist and former jury consultant whose plan provides an outdated diet combined with separate supplement packs for apple-shaped and pear-shaped individuals (with little justification for the difference in supplemention). Dr. Phil's approach is old-fashioned psychology with a strong tone of individual responsibility. Don't get me wrong. I think personal responsibility and willpower are important, but you have to know how to get there. Studies have shown that in smoking cessation you can tell people to stop smoking with some effectiveness. However, you can't just tell people they need to lose weight—you have to show them how. Basically, after telling you why your fat is your fault, Dr. Phil says, "Just get over it!"

If you have tried these diets or decided they were not for you, get ready for a simple, real-world diet that works. You can't do just one thing. Eliminating sugar and fruits, downing huge pieces of red meat, or cutting out all fats is not only impossible, but not necessary. The L.A. Shape Diet allows you to customize your plan according to your protein needs, your calorie needs, your target weight, and your food preferences and weaknesses. It allows you to choose what you will change in your diet and lifestyle.

Your Trigger Foods and Snack Defenses

You first need to identify the wrong foods you are eating. Some of these foods have a hold on you, and you can't control your consumption. Have you ever eaten just one chocolate chip cookie when a whole bag was open and available—and you weren't even especially hungry? This is a luxury that humans have developed just in the last one hundred years or so. The food industry calls this behavior "snacking," and has developed thousands of snack foods to encourage us to indulge in it. There is nothing wrong with eating five or six times a day if you are hungry and eat the right foods. The kind of behavior I'm talking about is eating when you have an urge or craving, without real hunger. Since you are not hungry, foods have to appeal to your taste buds or you won't spend the money to buy them. Fast-food french fries made from the Russett Burbank potato are fried in hydrogenated vegetable oils with added beef flavorings, and their smell draws you into the restaurant. But the real moneymaker is not the french fries and burgers, but the colas and other soft drinks, which have a 13,000 percent profit margin. An 8-ounce cola contains 150 calories, so at 32 ounces (a commonly offered size) you are taking in 600 calories. If those calories aren't enough, you can get another 800 calories for only 39 cents more by "supersizing" your fast-food meal. As one food industry CEO once told me, "People don't come to our products looking for health." I'll say!

In the list below you will find some snack foods and some meal choices that I have classified as Trigger Foods. Think of how often you eat these foods when you are not really hungry. In Step 4, you'll learn how to eliminate the urges to eat these foods by changing your behaviors.

Trigger Foods are the foods people tell you they "love," but it is actually a dysfunctional love/hate relationship. They make you feel good while you eat them, and then you feel guilty, knowing they will lead to weight gain. You may make all kinds of excuses as to why you were entitled to eat unconsciously just this once, or you may not even be aware of how much you have eaten. I don't want to take your doughnuts away, I want *you* to put them away. If you have ever started munching chips, nuts, or bread, only to notice that they were all gone, you know what I mean.

My patients have one of three common reactions on reviewing the Trigger Food list. Most people acknowledge which foods are a problem and go to work on those. Some people tell me I just described their whole diet; they have a lot of work to do. Others tell me they eat none of these foods and still cannot lose weight. These individuals have a low metabolic rate due to a low lean body mass, which I will explain later on in this chapter. For now, look at the list below and check off your personal Trigger Foods. While these are the most common ones, you may have other personal Trigger Foods that are not on this list.

Trigger Foods

- **NUTS**
- **CHEESE AND PIZZA**
- **FULL-FAT SALAD DRESSINGS**
- **MAYONNAISE, MARGARINE, AND BUTTER**
- **FATTY RED MEATS AND FATTY FISH**
- **BEANS, RICE, POTATOES, PASTA, CRACKERS, CHIPS, AND BREADS**
- **FROZEN YOGURT, ICE CREAM, CAKES, AND PASTRIES**
- **COLAS AND JUICES**
- **HARD LIQUOR, MIXED DRINKS, AND BEER**

Trigger Foods

You can prepare to change your eating habits for life by controlling your personal Trigger Food habits and the hidden calorie foods that may be sabotaging your efforts to lose weight. Pick the ones that apply to you, and begin to make these changes in your diet now and for the rest of your life.

Keep this short list in your head or on your refrigerator door where you will see it if you are looking around for food in the kitchen.

NUTS

Peanuts are fine as a flavor enhancer in a cooked dish, but by the handful, watch out. There is no end, especially when your baseball team is losing. Eating nuts as a snack is a portion-control and calorie issue with a cup of nuts containing over 800 calories.

CHEESE AND PIZZA

Are you a cheese lover? One slice of full-fat cheese has 140 calories per slice, and even nonfat cheese provides 80 calories per slice. Hard cheese has up to 80 percent fat. That can add up quickly if you are burning only 1,200 calories per day. Pizza is a food group unto itself. Most pizzas contain oil in their refined-flour crusts. Most have cheese on top, as well as some high-fat sausage and pepperoni, and some even have cheese stuffed in the crust, so the calories add up fast! *Try zucchini, spaghetti squash, or a high-fiber whole-wheat pasta with tomato sauce instead.*

SALAD DRESSING

Both creamy and oil-based salad dressings provide, on average, 150 calories and 10 to 20 grams of fat per ounce, not to mention added sugar. So, avoid all dressings, including so-called low-fat varieties. Olive oil is a healthy fat, but it contains the same calories per tablespoon as butter or margarine, so go easy.

Try dressing your salads simply with balsamic vinegar, rice vinegar, or wine vinegar instead, or use the salad dressing recipes in Step 3. Make your salad tasty with spinach and other dark green lettuces, tomatoes, alfalfa sprouts, green pepper, and other vegetables so that you don't depend on the dressing to carry the taste.

MAYONNAISE, MARGARINE, AND BUTTER

So-called nonfat margarine actually provides 100 percent of its calories from fat, since it is like the regular margarine—just diluted. The USDA (U.S. Department of Agriculture) has ruled that if a serving of margarine has less than ½ gram of fat, it can be called nonfat. This is the only place in mathematics in which you can round down from 0.5 to zero. In the Appendix, I compare good fats and bad fats, but they all have 120 calories per tablespoon including mayonnaise, margarine, and butter.

Try eating high-fiber bread with just a thin layer of fruit jam, or if you are having a sandwich, use mustard or ketchup instead of mayonnaise.

FATTY RED MEATS AND FATTY FISH

One of the easiest places to reduce a lot of calories is fatty red meats and fatty fish. Fatty cuts of red meat include veal, beef, pork, and lamb. A piece of prime rib contains 1,500 calories and 50 grams of saturated fat, which is all the calories and more fat than most five-foot-tall women need for a whole day. And I'm sorry to have to tell you, but pork is not the other white meat! You can choose to eat some lean cuts of red meat—including filet mignon, top sirloin, or flank steak—up to once a week or not at all; it's your choice. Be careful on portion sizes of red meat, especially in restaurants. Try to eat 3 to 6 ounces of lean red meat. Three ounces is about the size of the palm of your hand. *Substitute skinless white meat of chicken or white meat of turkey for red meat.* If it will help, put steak sauce on chicken and pretend it's red meat. Be careful—*dark poultry meat is higher in fat than white meat and can have as much fat as some cuts of red meat.*

Farm-raised salmon, trout, and catfish are higher in calories and fat than ocean-caught fish, such as tuna and halibut, because farmed fish get very little exercise and don't feed on the healthy fish and algae that the ocean-caught fish do. While the content of so-called good fat (see the Appendix for a complete explanation) is similar in farmed and ocean-caught salmon, the farmed variety have twice as much "bad fat" in addition to the "good fat." Farmed salmon is the marbled steak of the fish world, with more than 800 calories in an 8-ounce serving. *Substitute halibut, cod, sole, canned white tuna packed in water, orange roughy, red snapper, or shark. Shrimp, scallops, lobster, and crab are also low in fat. Avoid the small bay shrimp, swordfish, and Lake Superior whitefish, which are higher in mercury than other fish.*

BEANS, RICE, POTATOES, PASTA, CRACKERS, CHIPS, AND BREADS

While you may think that some of these foods are healthy, you need to know that a cup of rice, beans, pasta, or potatoes has 250 calories compared to only 40 calories or less for a cup of most vegetables. *Order a double portion of vegetables in the restaurant and skip the mashed potatoes or rice on your dinner plate.* It's an easy way to cut out over 200 calories. Ask your waiter not to bring chips or bread to the table before your meal. You may eat 550 calories in a basket of chips or 320 calories in a bagel or several slices of bread. *Eat only one slice of high-fiber bread, which has 3 to 5 grams of fiber in about 70 calories, and you will get full faster—or skip the bread altogether.* You need only three servings per day of high-fiber whole-grain foods. Read the label carefully; there are no label standards for "whole grain."

Potato chips, french fries, snack crackers, and pretzels are just fine when viewed in the abstract. However, when you look at how they are eaten by most Americans, you're talking about hundreds of extra calories. Only twenty potato chips can contain 150 calories. That means forty chips have 300 calories, and so on—to even more frightening calorie totals. An extra 500 calories per day—leading to a pound of weight gain per week—is easy to consume without even blinking. An alternative healthy snack substitute for potato chips is roasted soy nuts, which provide about 100 calories per 1-ounce serving and help with salty cravings.

FROZEN YOGURT, ICE CREAM, CAKES, AND PASTRIES

These treats add lots of extra calories from fat and sugar. Even the fat-free versions pack in many extra calories, because they are loaded with sugar and can be loaded with calories. Instead, *have a piece of fruit, or drizzle chocolate syrup on fresh strawberries, bananas, pineapple, or other fruit to satisfy your sweet tooth.* Or try one of the new "light-and-fit" yogurts with more protein, or fruit sorbet (but watch the sugar).

SOFT DRINKS AND JUICES

As mentioned earlier, 8 ounces (less than a can) of soda has 150 calories, and 32 ounces has 600! *While diet colas and soft drinks are all right, they do maintain the habit of drinking soft drinks, so you are not actually breaking a habit. Drink plain or sparkling water with a slice of lemon or lime.*

Fruit juices may sound healthy, but if you drink a 16-ounce bottle that's labeled 130 calories, you are really consuming 260 calories—a 130-calorie serving is only 8 ounces, or half the bottle. The USDA says that anything over 12 ounces is two servings, so the manufacturers get to put a lower number of calories on the label, assuming (often correctly) that you're not going to look at the serving size. You practically need a degree in nutrition to uncover these deceptions. *Have a piece of fruit instead of fruit juice (you'll be getting valuable fiber as well), or flavor water with small amounts of 100 percent juice.*

HARD LIQUOR, MIXED DRINKS, AND BEER

A glass of beer contains 220 calories and is a refined grain, as are hard liquors, including scotch, gin, and whiskey. Among mixed drinks, the margarita has the most calories, at 350 per average serving. A good alternative in a social situation is carbonated water and lime instead of a mixed drink, or one small glass of red wine, which contains healthy resveratrol and only about 80 calories. If you have to have a beer, have one light beer or ultra-light beer (containing 70 to 110 calories).

Think about the calorie costs of your Trigger Food habits listed in the following chart. How many calories could you save by eating a vegetable or fruit instead? Remember that the average woman needs only 1,500 calories per day, and the average man needs only 2,100 calories per day.

So, what is so hard about controlling Trigger Foods? Well, humans are creatures of habit. If you eat Trigger Foods, they have a strong hold on you personally. What a Trigger Food is for you may not be the same one for another person. It will take time and patience to change yourself. You may have managed to stop smoking, but this is harder. In fact, there is nothing harder, but I will try to make it easier by asking you to make simple changes whenever possible.

You may choose not to stop eating Trigger Foods altogether. But at the very least I will make you think before you eat, and choose how much you want to eat. You will set your own limits—it's up to you.

Personalizing Your Program

CALORIES AND FAT IN TYPICAL TRIGGER FOODS

Food item	Portion	Calories	Fat grams and teaspoons of fat
Soft drink	20-ounce bottle	250	0
Peanuts	1 cup	835	71 grams / 14 teaspoons
BBQ potato chips	7-ounce bag	970	64 grams / 13 teaspoons
Corn chips	7-ounce bag	1,065	66 grams / 13 teaspoons
French fries	40 strips	630	33 grams / 7 teaspoons
Cheese and Ritz crackers	2 ounces cheese + 12 crackers	410	28 grams / 6 teaspoons
Pizza, stuffed crust, super supreme	2 slices	1020	52 grams / 10 teaspoons
Carrot cake with icing	1 average slice	485	29 grams / 6 teaspoons
Chocolate chip cookies	6 small	350	16 grams / 3 teaspoons
Apple pie	1 average slice	410	19 grams / 4 teaspoons
Pretzels	25 twists	570	5 grams / 1 teaspoon
Peanut butter and crackers	9 sandwiches	300	15 grams / 3 teaspoons
Bagel and cream cheese	Medium-size bagel + 2 tablespoons cream cheese	400	10 grams / 2 teaspoons
Blueberry muffin	1 large	410	10 grams / 2 teaspoons
Typical candy bar	3 ounce bar	465	32 grams / $6\frac{1}{2}$ teaspoons
Ice cream	1 cup	350	24 grams / 5 teaspoons
Granola bars	2	325	18 grams / $3\frac{1}{2}$ teaspoons
Cream-filled doughnut	1	310	21 grams / 4 teaspoons

Some Trigger Foods taste good because added fat amplifies their sweet taste. So you may think of a candy bar as a sweet, but it is really a sweet-fat combination, adding lots of extra calories. And taste is not the only hold they have on you. Food advertising applies psychology to make you want to eat these foods so as to be or feel a certain way. Steak makes you strong. Ice cream makes you happy. Chocolate. . . . let's not go there. You can't eat just one potato chip. A caramel-colored soft drink sweetened with corn syrup is either the real thing or the drink of a new generation. These subconscious messages are not accidents; they are carefully researched by teams of workers interviewing people like you to see how best to get inside your head. These focus groups and taste testers have enabled the cola makers to zero in on the perfect amount of sweetener to appeal to most people (about 10.5 percent sugar by weight). Then food scientists go to work to see how to deliver the taste experience using high-fructose corn syrup, vegetable oil, and artificial colors and flavors to keep the costs down and the profits up. All the while they are selling more food (if you can call it that) containing more calories to people like you and me who are simply trying to get healthier or lose a few pounds so that they can fit into their clothes again.

Your Target Weight, Target Shape, and Body Fat

Finding the right target weight and shape for you personally is critical. Many studies have demonstrated that individuals tend to want to weigh much less than would be medically desirable based on percent body fat. Men should have between 15 and 20 percent body fat, while women should have between 22 and 28 percent body fat. Young women up to about age 20 who are athletic should have 15 to 20 percent body fat, and certain athletes like college basketball or track athletes with very high muscle mass can have as little as 5 percent body fat (and typically have 8 to 10 percent body fat). Wrestlers who try to lose weight aggressively to get into a lower weight category are legally limited to having at least 5 percent body fat, and that is generally regarded as an absolute minimum for safety. What's important to you, however, is not to reach the minimum level but rather aim for a range that's reasonable for you.

Finding Your Reasonable Target Weight and Best Shape

At a reasonable target weight, you will have enough protein in your muscles and heart to be healthy. At this reasonable target weight, you will also have a healthy shape that is just right for you. If you try to lose weight below a target weight estimated by a so-called ideal fat percentage, you will lose protein from your muscles and your heart. Then your shape won't look so wonderful, as your arms and legs lose muscle and get flabby.

A famous photographer who was given the assignment to do the bathing suit issue for *Sports Illustrated* each year took a strong position on which girls would be selected for the annual swimsuit issue. Unlike other fashion photographers, she refused to photograph Twiggy-type models who were too thin and had too little muscle. Instead, she insisted that her models have some muscles showing along with their curves, and that they look fit and healthy. Her stand on this issue was one of the first steps toward making a desirable female shape more realistic. There are lots of successful women in business and entertainment today who have all kinds of body shapes, from curvy hips and muscular thighs to more muscle in their shoulders. While many women strive to be tiny, men want to be big with lots of bulging muscles. Shape is less of an obsession with men, but they also need to be realistic about their potential best body shape. There are no best shapes other than the one you achieve personally—and you *can* achieve it, no matter where you are starting from. The key is to be happy with who you are and to embrace and love your best shape.

Your Calorie Needs and Predicted Rate of Weight Loss

I can estimate your calorie needs in several ways. The easiest way is simply to measure how much fat and lean you have. Lean tissues burn on average about 14 calories per pound per day at rest. So, a woman with 100 pounds of lean mass will burn 1,400 calories per day at rest and her husband, with 150 pounds of lean mass, will burn 2,100 calories per day at rest. That means that if they eat the same foods, she will gain 75 pounds in a year, while he will stay at the same weight. Put another way, if they both go on a diet of 1,200 calories per day, he will lose about 6 pounds a month and she will lose only about 2 pounds, assuming their activity levels and exercise burn the same number of calories.

The number of calories you burn at any time during the day will vary depending on whether you are sleeping, working on a computer, or exercising. Resting metabolism is the scientific term for the number of calories you burn lying down in bed the first thing in the morning. This is close to the average for the whole day and accounts for about 75 percent of all the calories you burn each day. You burn fewer calories in the middle of the night and up to 25 percent more calories per day through exercise, but I have found that the number of calories you burn at rest or your resting metabolism is the best indicator of how much weight you will lose on a diet.

You can't change your metabolism easily, but the most effective way to raise your metabolism is by building muscle. Build ten extra pounds of muscle, and now you will burn another 140 calories per day. Exercise for a half an hour on a treadmill and you might burn 200 calories. Eat that burger, fries, and a shake, and you just had 1,300 calories. In the Appendix, I have included a section with the latest science on how to build muscle most effectively.

So you see, the mathematics of weight loss is just not fair—or is it? Our bodies are simply designed not to lose weight. For the last 50,000 years of human history, that is exactly what we needed. But our genome has not been able to adapt our metabolism to burn the extra calories from home-delivered pizza or cream-filled doughnuts. You can't afford to wait for evolution, which could take a few million years, so what can you do right now?

Personalizing Your Protein Needs—The Magic 29 Percent

Your lean body mass determines how much protein you need each day, and it's about twice what was recommended by government advisory groups until recently, when the Institute of Medicine broadened their recommendation to any level of protein between 10 and 35 percent. This was done largely to recognize the new higher-protein diets while also including low-protein and low-fat diets such as the original Pritikin diet at 15 percent protein calories.

The Zone diet and Atkins high-protein diet recommend that 30 to 35 percent of calories come from protein along with either 30 percent or 59 percent fat calories. My recommendation is 29 percent of total calories from protein, which strangely enough, is, not that different from what

Atkins and the Zone recommend. I came to this 29 percent number for an entirely different reason—and The L.A. Shape Diet plan has less fat and more fruits and vegetables, as well as many other differences from the earlier diets.

Twenty-nine percent is a little abstract when it comes to deciding how much protein you need to eat each day. What's most important is to calculate how many grams of protein you need each day as the base of your diet. The most accurate way to determine this number is to calculate your lean body mass, which includes everything in your body that isn't fat, such as muscle, bone, organs, and skin. This number of pounds is about the number of grams of protein you need each day.

As your lean body mass increases, so does the number of calories you burn each day at rest. Each pound of lean body mass burns 14 calories per day at rest. For example, a woman burning 1,400 calories per day at rest (with 100 pounds of lean body mass) needs 100 grams of protein.

$$100 \text{ pounds of lean body mass} \times 14 \text{ calories per pound} = 1,400 \text{ calories per day}$$

A man burning 2,100 calories per day at rest (with 150 pounds of lean body mass) needs 150 grams of protein.

$$150 \text{ pounds of lean body mass} \times 14 \text{ calories per pound} = 2,100 \text{ calories per day}$$

In each case, the calories from protein at 4 calories per gram work out to be about 29 percent of resting calorie needs. For example, 100 pounds of lean mass translates into 1,400 calories per day at rest. One hundred grams of protein contains 400 calories. If you divide 400 calories by 1,400 calories, you get 29 percent. If you divide 600 calories from 150 grams of dietary protein by 2,100 calories, you get the same number. This rule works for any number of calories burned and so becomes the magic 29 percent.

The most accurate and practical way to determine your lean body mass is with a bioelectrical impedance meter, which measures both fat and lean. If you don't have access to such a meter through your doctor, nutritionist, or personal weight counselor, then the next two tables will help you estimate your daily protein target without making any specialized measurements such as bioelectrical impedance analysis. For more information about methods of body composition and bioelectrical impedance analysis, see the Appendix.

First, use your height and weight to find your Body Mass Index (BMI) in the following table, on page 47.

Then, using your BMI and your height, find your protein target estimate in the tables on pages 48 and 49. Round up to the next 25-gram unit of protein. So, if your estimated protein target is 112 grams, round up to 125—and consume 125 grams of protein per day. If your estimated protein target is 145, consume 150 grams of protein per day. And so on.

DETERMINING YOUR BODY MASS INDEX

BMI kg/m^2 Height	19	20	21	22	23	24	25	26	27	28	29	30	31	32	33	34	35	36	37	38	39	40
58	91	96	100	105	110	115	119	124	129	134	138	143	148	153	158	162	167	172	177	181	186	191
59	94	99	104	109	114	119	124	128	133	138	143	148	153	158	163	168	173	178	183	188	193	198
60	97	102	107	112	118	123	128	133	138	143	148	153	158	163	168	174	179	184	189	194	199	204
61	100	106	111	116	122	127	132	137	143	148	153	158	164	169	174	180	185	190	195	201	206	211
62	104	109	115	120	126	131	136	142	147	153	158	164	169	175	180	186	191	196	202	207	213	218
63	107	113	118	124	130	135	141	146	152	158	163	169	175	180	186	191	197	203	208	214	220	225
64	110	116	122	128	134	140	145	151	157	163	169	174	180	186	192	197	204	209	215	221	227	232
65	114	120	126	132	138	144	150	156	162	168	174	180	186	192	198	204	210	216	222	228	234	240
66	118	124	130	136	142	148	155	161	167	173	179	186	192	198	204	210	216	223	229	235	241	247
67	121	127	134	140	146	153	159	166	172	178	185	191	198	204	211	217	223	230	236	242	249	255
68	125	131	138	144	151	158	164	171	177	184	190	197	203	210	216	223	230	236	243	249	256	262
69	128	135	142	149	155	162	169	176	182	189	196	203	209	216	223	230	236	243	250	257	263	270
70	132	139	146	153	160	167	174	181	188	195	202	207	216	222	229	236	243	250	257	264	271	278
71	136	143	150	157	165	172	179	186	193	200	208	215	222	229	236	243	250	257	265	272	279	286
72	140	147	154	162	169	177	184	191	199	206	213	221	228	235	242	250	258	265	272	279	287	294
73	144	151	159	166	174	182	189	197	204	212	219	227	235	242	250	257	265	272	280	288	295	302
74	148	155	163	171	179	186	194	202	210	218	225	233	241	249	256	264	272	280	287	295	303	311
75	152	160	168	176	184	192	200	208	216	224	232	240	248	256	264	272	279	287	295	303	311	319
76	156	164	172	180	189	197	205	213	221	230	238	246	254	263	271	279	287	296	304	312	320	328

Source: National Heart, Lung and Blood Institute

The table above already includes the results of the math and metric conversions to determine BMI. To use the table, find your height in the left-hand column. Move across the row to your weight. The number at the top of the column in which you find your weight is the BMI for your height and weight.

ESTIMATED PROTEIN TARGET INTAKE FOR WOMEN (GRAMS PER DAY)

Height	Body Mass Index (BMI)												
	19	20	21	22	23	24	25	26	27	28	29	30	31
4'10"–5'0"	79	81	81	84	86	86	87	88	91	91	92	94	96
5'1"–5'4"	91	95	97	98	99	101	102	103	106	107	109	109	112
5'5"–5'8"	105	107	110	110	113	114	117	119	122	122	123	127	131
5'9"–6'0"	118	120	122	125	127	129	131	133	135	138	140	142	144

Height	Body Mass Index (BMI)								
	32	33	34	35	36	37	38	39	40
4'10"–5'0"	97	99	99	101	102	105	105	107	108
5'1"–5'4"	114	116	118	120	121	122	124	127	128
5'5"–5'8"	130	131	134	135	138	140	142	143	145
5'9"–6'0"	146	149	151	153	154	156	158	161	163

ESTIMATED PROTEIN TARGET INTAKE FOR MEN (GRAMS PER DAY)

Height	Body Mass Index (BMI)												
	19	20	21	22	23	24	25	26	27	28	29	30	31
5'1"–5'4"	107	109	111	112	114	117	117	118	120	122	123	124	127
5'5"–5'8"	122	123	124	127	129	131	132	135	136	139	140	143	144
5'9"–6'0"	135	138	140	143	144	147	150	152	154	156	157	160	162
6'1"–6'4"	151	155	157	158	162	165	166	168	172	174	176	179	182

Height	Body Mass Index (BMI)								
	32	33	34	35	36	37	38	39	40
5'1"–5'4"	129	130	132	134	135	136	139	141	142
5'5"–5'8"	145	147	150	152	156	156	157	160	161
5'9"–6'0"	164	166	168	171	173	175	177	178	180
6'1"–6'4"	184	187	187	190	194	196	198	201	202

Now that you know how much protein to eat, select the high-protein/low-fat foods that you prefer from the following table, including lean meat, chicken, fish, seafood, egg whites, nonfat dairy products, and soy meat substitutes. All these proteins are high quality, meaning that they contain the proper mix of amino acid building blocks your body needs for good health. You can choose a vegetarian diet using soy protein, which is high-quality protein, or you can select high-quality animal proteins such as egg whites, cottage cheese, and lean meats. If you want to eat both, I usually recommend that half the units come from animal sources and half from vegetarian foods for best health results, based on some scientific studies in animals that highlight the different amino acids found in animal and vegetable proteins.

PROTEIN FOODS IN UNITS OF ABOUT 25 GRAMS EACH

Food Item	One Unit	Calories	Protein (gm)
Breakfast			
Egg whites	7 whites	115	25
Nonfat cottage cheese	1 cup	140	28
Flavored soy protein meal replacement and nonfat milk	1 serving flavored soy protein and 1 cup nonfat milk	180–200 (varies)	19–25 (varies)
Vegetarian			
Soy Canadian bacon	4 slices	80	21 (varies)
Plain soy protein powder	1 ounce	110	20–25
Soy nugget cereal	½ cup	140	25 (varies)
Flavored soy protein meal replacement and soy milk	1 serving flavored soy protein and 1 cup soy milk	180–200 (varies)	19–25 (varies)

The L.A. Shape Diet

Food Item	One Unit	Calories	Protein (gm)
Lunch and Dinner			
Turkey breast	3 ounces, cooked weight	135	25
Chicken breast	3 ounces, cooked weight	140	25
Lean red meat	3 ounces, cooked weight	145–160	25
Ocean-caught fish (salmon, tuna, sea bass)	4 ounces, cooked weight	130–170	25–31
Shrimp, crab, lobster	4 ounces, cooked weight	120	22–24
Tuna	4 ounces, water pack	145	27
Scallops	4 ounces, cooked weight	135	25
Egg whites	7 whites	115	25
Nonfat cottage cheese	1 cup	140	28
Vegetarian			
Plain soy protein powder	1 ounce	110	20–25
Soy hot dog	2 links	110	22 (varies)
Soy "ground round"	¾ cup	120	24 (varies)
Soy burgers	2 patties	160	26 (varies)
Tofu, firm	½ cup	180	20 (varies)

The Rest of the Diet

Plants make sugars, proteins, and fats that they need for fuel, and we eat these as food for calories. Plants also make thousands of phytochemicals that have other functions such as regulating plant growth, attracting helpful bacteria, or fighting off pests. While these phytochemicals were developed by plants for their own purposes, they have profound effects on our bodies by acting as antioxidants in the cells of our bodies and having specific effects on health.

Modern medicine has concentrated and purified phytochemicals in order to make drugs from plants. In fact, two-thirds of all drugs come from plants. A recent blockbuster example is Taxol, derived from the bark of the yew tree, which has become a very effective anti-cancer drug. In lower doses, many such chemicals may be able to prevent some of the most common diseases associated with aging, including cancer. Phytochemicals are found as families of related chemicals rather than as the purified crystals found in the medicines developed by the drug industry.

The colors in fruits and vegetables are related to the phytochemical families they contain. The red color of tomatoes comes from a family of compounds, including lycopene (the best known), phytoene, phytofluene, vitamin E, and vitamin C. The lycopene localizes in the prostate glands of men, where increasing scientific evidence points to a role in cancer prevention. The orange color in carrots, pumpkins, and butternut squash comes from beta-carotene, which is converted to vitamin A for maintaining healthy vision and for cancer prevention. The yellow-green chemical lutein, which occurs together with zeaxanthin in many plants, such as spinach and other green leafy vegetables, localizes in the back of the eye in the part of the retina, where the most light is concentrated. There is evidence that lutein may help prevent macular degeneration, the most common cause of age-related blindness. The purple color of blueberries represents families of chemicals that may prevent age-related memory loss. The chart on page 54 lists the colors of the fruits and vegetables together with the phytochemicals they contain; it will be clear why I recommend eating seven servings every day. There are supplements that can provide these phytochemicals in tablet or capsule form if you don't manage to get in all seven servings every day.

Colorful fruits and vegetables have healthy carbohydrates that will not cause you to gain weight, no matter what you read in those books that told you carrots and bananas were fattening. No fruits or vegetables are fattening, except those that are starchy such as beans and potatoes—and they are not in the recommended lists of fruits and vegetables.

Servings can be hard to understand. The official definition of a serving is ½ a cup of cooked vegetable or fruit, but a whole cup of raw vegetables. We have simplified most of the tables to indicate 1 cup as a portion size so as to remove some of this confusion. The healthy restaurant dinner I compared to an unhealthy dinner on page 95 would give you five servings of fruits and vegetables just in that one meal. It is not surprising, therefore, that the average intake of fruits and vegetables is a pound (or about seven servings) in countries where people have really healthy diets. If you want to fill up at dinner and eat more to weigh less, then concentrate on vegetables such as spinach rather than on fruits. I like to have a cup of cooked spinach (two servings) topped with tomato sauce (½ cup, or one serving) for a total of only 90 calories (40 for the spinach and 50 for the tomato sauce)—and this means I eat from two color groups at the same time. At dessert, how about some frozen or fresh blueberries? A half cup gives you the additional benefits of purple-colored phytochemicals (called anthocyanins) found in this great fruit. They are purple because their chemical structure makes them absorb visible light except for the blue-purple part of the rainbow. Most restaurants will make you a dessert bowl of mixed fruit, such as strawberries, raspberries, or melons in season.

Fruits and vegetables are also great sources of fiber. Your goal for each day is 25 grams of fiber, which can come from five servings of fruits or vegetables with 5 grams of fiber per serving. The list that follows shows in

Personalizing Your Program

Color	Fruits and Vegetables	Main Phytonutrients and Their Benefits
Red	Tomatoes, tomato soup, juices or sauces, and pink grapefruit or watermelon	**Lycopene** is one of the most potent free radical scavengers in nature. It may reduce the risk of heart and lung disease, as well as prostate cancer.
Red/Purple	Red grapes, blueberries, blackberries, cherries, plums, prunes, raspberries, strawberries, red apples	**Anthocyanins** are powerful anti-oxidants that strengthen skin and other tissues, tendons, and ligaments. They may help with age-related declines in mental function.
Orange	Apricots, acorn and winter squash, butternut and yellow squash, carrots, mangoes, cantaloupes, pumpkin, sweet potatoes	**Alpha and Beta Carotene** are carotenoids and very effective antioxidants. They protect against cancer by preventing oxidative damage, and promote vision by conversion to vitamin A.
Orange/Yellow	Clementines, Mandarin oranges, oranges and orange juice, peaches, pineapple and pineapple juice, nectarines, papayas, tangerines, tangelos	The rinds of citrus fruit contain limonene and other chemicals that have some anticancer effects. The vitamin C and flavonoids are included in a rich matrix in whole fruits.
Yellow/Green	Spinach, avocado, dark green lettuces, green and yellow peppers, green beans, kale, mustard greens, green peas, honeydew melon, yellow corn	**Lutein and zeaxanthin** are pigments that become concentrated in the retina, where they help reduce the risk of cataracts and age-related macular degeneration.
Green	Broccoli and broccoli sprouts, Bok Choy, Brussels sprouts, cabbage, Chinese cabbage, kale	**Sulforaphane, isothiocyanate, and indoles** fight numerous diseases by stimulating formation of enzymes that can eliminate toxic drugs and carcinogens from the body.
White/Green	Asparagus, celery, chives, endive, garlic, leeks, mushrooms, pearl onions, pears, shallots	**Allyl sulfides** are compounds that give garlic and onions their odor but also can promote blood vessel health. **Quercetin** is a flavonoid with anticancer potential as well.

boldface type those fruits and vegetables that contain 5 or more grams of fiber per serving. Your best bet is to select up to five servings providing 5 or more grams of fiber that you can eat on a regular basis so that you can be sure to get your 25 grams of fiber. If you can only eat three servings, then you need 10 grams of a fiber supplement. The latest versions of these supplements contain fructooligosaccharides, guar gum, and other soluble fibers. You can mix them with your coffee or put them into your protein shake in the morning without affecting the taste at all. High-fiber cereals are another way to get fiber into your diet, but be careful. In the Appendix you'll find a list of the fiber, protein, and sugar content of common cereals. You'll need to choose carefully if you are going to include cereals in your diet. I think the Empowering Shake every morning is a great way to get your L.A. Shape and keep it, but if you want cereal once in a while, just read the list carefully.

COLOR GROUPS OF FRUITS AND VEGETABLES

(Women and men: Choose at least *one* item from each color group every day.)

Red

Food Item	Portion	Calories	Fiber (grams)
Tomato juice	1 cup	40	1
Tomato sauce/purée	**1 cup**	**100**	**5**
Tomato soup, made with water	1 cup	85	0
Tomato vegetable juice	1 cup	45	2
Tomatoes, cooked	1 cup	70	3
Tomatoes, raw	1 large	40	2
Watermelon	1 cup balls	50	1

COLOR GROUPS OF FRUITS AND VEGETABLES (*CONTINUED*)

Red/Purple

Food Item	Portion	Calories	Fiber (grams)
Beets, cooked	1 cup	75	3
Blackberries	**1 cup**	**75**	**8**
Blueberries	**1 cup**	**110**	**5**
Eggplant, cooked	**2 cups**	**60**	**5**
Pomegranate	1 medium	120	1
Plums	3 small	100	3
Raspberries	**1 cup**	**100**	**8**
Red apple	1 medium	100	4
Red cabbage, cooked	**2 cups**	**60**	**6**
Red pepper	1 large	45	3
Red wine	4-ounce glass	80	0
Strawberries	**1½ cups, sliced**	**75**	**6**

Orange

Food Item	Portion	Calories	Fiber (grams)
Acorn squash, baked	**1 cup**	**85**	**6**
Apricot	5 whole	85	4
Cantaloupe	½ medium	80	2
Carrots, cooked	1 cup	70	5
Carrots, raw	**3 medium**	**75**	**6**
Mango	½ large	80	3
Pumpkin, cooked	1 cup	50	3
Winter squash, baked	**1 cup**	**70**	**7**

Orange/Yellow

Food Item	Portion	Calories	Fiber (grams)
Nectarine	1 large	70	2
Orange	1 large	85	4
Papaya	½ large	75	3

Food Item	Portion	Calories	Fiber (grams)
Peach	1 large	70	3
Pineapple	1 cup, diced	75	2
Tangerine	**2 medium**	**85**	**5**
Yellow grapefruit	1 fruit	75	2

Yellow/Green

Food Item	Portion	Calories	Fiber (grams)
Avocado	$\frac{1}{4}$ average fruit	80	2
Banana	1 average	90	2
Collard greens, cooked	**2 cups**	**100**	**10**
Cucumber	1 average	40	2
Green beans, cooked	**2 cups**	**85**	**8**
Green pepper	1 large	45	3
Honeydew	$\frac{1}{4}$ large melon	100	2
Kiwi	1 large	55	3
Mustard greens, cooked	**2 cups**	**40**	**6**
Romaine lettuce	4 cups	30	4
Spinach, cooked	**2 cups**	**80**	**8**
Spinach, raw	4 cups	30	4
Turnip greens, cooked	**2 cups**	**60**	**10**
Yellow pepper	1 large	50	2
Zucchini with skin, cooked	**2 cups**	**60**	**5**

Green

Food Item	Portion	Calories	Fiber (grams)
Broccoli, cooked	**2 cups**	**85**	**9**
Brussels sprouts	1 cup	60	4
Cabbage, cooked	**2 cups**	**70**	**8**
Cabbage, raw	2 cups	40	4
Cauliflower, cooked	**2 cups**	**55**	**6**
Chinese cabbage, cooked	**2 cups**	**40**	**5**

Personalizing Your Program

Food Item	Portion	Calories	Fiber (grams)
Kale, cooked	**2 cups**	**70**	**5**
Swiss chard	**2 cups**	**70**	**7**
White/Green			

Food Item	Portion	Calories	Fiber (grams)
Artichoke	**1 medium**	**60**	**6**
Asparagus	18 spears	60	4
Celery	3 large stalks	30	3
Chives	2 tablespoons	2	0
Endive, raw	**½ head**	**45**	**8**
Garlic	1 clove	5	0
Leeks, cooked	1 medium	40	1
Mushrooms, cooked	1 cup	40	3
Onion	1 large	60	3

How much fiber could you get from your fruits and vegetables in one day? Use the charts above to plan your typical days. You can also use these to help complete your food diary given in the Appendix.

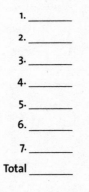

1. _____
2. _____
3. _____
4. _____
5. _____
6. _____
7. _____
Total _____

Starches and Grains

Fiber is found both in the fruits and vegetables listed in the preceding tables and in the grains discussed in this section. If you are not getting the recommended 25 grams of fiber from your fruits and vegetables, the remainder of your fiber can come from whole grains or a fiber supplement. You must also worry about total calories, even with whole grains. Eat carbohydrates in whole grains in very limited amounts. One slice of whole grain bread can contain 100 calories. Beans, rice, lentils, and other starchy vegetables have 200 to 250 calories per cup, compared to 40 calories per cup of spinach or broccoli. Corn and peas are included even though they have 140 to 150 calories per cup. They have fewer calories per cup than beans, but more than most vegetables. So they should be eaten in small servings, which is why I indicate the ½ cup serving size in the following table even though the official USDA serving size is 1 cup. All of the servings are designed to be in the same calorie range. However, don't fool yourself. Is that really ½ cup of beans or are you eating a full cup or two and getting 250 to 500 calories? If you can't control your portions of these foods, skip them altogether.

This is a good place to review the difference between good carbohydrates and bad carbohydrates. As I have already said, eating no carbohydrates is impossible. Instead, I suggest you eat "good" carbohydrates, such as those from whole fruits and vegetables, instead of pretzels, potato chips, candy bars, and other snacks. Fruits and vegetables are calorie bargains, and they have other healthy properties. After saying how easy a "no carb" diet is at first, patients come back to me a year later saying that they just couldn't keep eliminating carbohydrates, validating my clinical experience and what is found in the scientific literature.

But do look carefully at your plate and cut down on grains such as white rice and pasta, and limit potatoes and beans whenever possible. Even whole grains have lots of calories per bite; eat them no more than one to three serv-

Starch/grain units (1 unit is between 60 and 140 calories; choose carefully)	Serving size	Calories	Fiber (grams)	Protein (grams)
Cooked beans	½ cup, cooked	115–140	5–7	7
Brown rice	½ cup, cooked	110	2	3
Lentils	½ cup, cooked	115	8	9
Green peas	½ cup	70	4	4
Corn	½ cup kernels or 1 ear	75	3	2
Sweet potato (yam)	½ cup, mashed	100	3	2
Bread, whole grain*	1 slice	60–100	2–3	3–5

*Check the food labels on every brand you buy, since there is no standard for whole grains. You should be able to find breads that meet these profiles at your grocery store. If not, ask your grocer to carry whole-grain breads, and in the meantime buy them in a natural foods store.

ings per day. Cutting back on grains will not hurt you while you are losing weight and is a great way to cut calories. If you find you are having a hard time maintaining your weight once you have lost it (this is the kind of problem few of my patients have but would like to have), then whole grains are a good way to keep your weight from dropping. Men with high calorie requirements will need whole grains to maintain their weight and their energy level.

The Fat Secret of "No-Carb" Diets

Beyond the filling effects of protein, the "no-carb" diets have a lot of fat. In fact, Atkins recommends an intake of 59 percent fat calories and only 5 percent carbohydrates. So what do you get when you put high fat and high protein together? The original Atkins diet. But people on Atkins don't eat this much fat. They tell me they are on a modified plan or the new Atkins plan devised in the few months before Dr. Atkins's tragic death from a fall on the ice in New York.

Since Atkins dieters are not able to bring themselves to eat all this fat, which they know is not healthy, instead of zero fat, they often develop an obsession with zero carbohydrates. In fact, they don't realize that the vegetables and salads on the modified Atkins diet contain carbohydrates, and they obsess over how many grams of carbohydrates are listed on protein bars. This has set off a war among the protein-bar makers to get to zero carbs, which is impossible. Instead, they have gone to substituting sugar alcohols for carbs, which your body breaks down to sugar just the same. The sugar alcohol is not recognized by the Food and Drug Administration as a necessary part of the nutrition label, where all carbohydrates are listed.

Since getting to zero carbs is nearly impossible, it is often a pointless effort and you could be spending your energy on building a healthy diet in other areas. But as with most theories, there is a grain of truth here. Carbohydrate cravings can alter brain chemistry and stimulate binge eating. If refined sugars and starches are triggers for you, then eliminate those from your diet. In Step 3, I give more detail on the refined carbohydrates that are most likely to stimulate craving. They are the ones that raise blood sugar and insulin more rapidly than other foods. However, total grams of carbohydrates and total calories in the food also count.

The Science Behind Carbohydrate Craving

In the 1970s and 1980s, Dr. Richard Wurtman and his wife, Judith, developed a behavioral concept called "carbohydrate craving," which you have probably experienced as "you can't eat just one." Some carbohydrates, such as refined sugars and starches, have a potent habit-forming effect by increasing the levels of blood insulin rapidly after you eat.

An increase in insulin drives many amino acids, the building blocks of protein, into the muscles, with the exception of tryptophan. As the tryptophan concentration is increased relative to other amino acids, it crosses the blood-brain barrier and interacts with a protein in the part of the brain that stimulates pleasure. The pleasure hormone (or neurochemical) is serotonin, and it can be made from tryptophan. Once you experience this pleasure, you want to repeat the behavior again. With so little pleasure in some people's lives, their carbohydrates become their friends, enabling them to get through the day.

Glycemic Index, Glycemic Load, and Calories

Years ago we simply talked about refined and complex carbohydrates. The refined carbohydrates were considered bad because they caused a rapid rise in blood sugar, which could trigger snacking through effects on brain chemistry. Then in the 1980s, Dr. David Jenkins of the University of Toronto developed the glycemic index (GI). To determine this, you calculate how much the blood sugar rises when a certain food is eaten over a period of several hours and compare it to the blood-sugar rise caused by a fixed dose of pure corn sugar (or dextrose). In practice, a chart is made of the values of blood sugar as it rises over time, and the dots are connected, creating a curve. The area under the curve of blood sugars, after the administration of a fixed number of calories of the test food, is calculated and compared to the area following the administration of the same number of calories of glucose in that person, which is given an arbitrary score of 100. The higher the number, the greater the blood sugar response and the greater the resulting emotional impact on sugar craving. So a low-GI food will cause a small rise, while a high-GI food will trigger a dramatic spike in blood sugar. A list of foods with their glycemic values is shown beginning on page 65. A GI of 55 or more is considered high, and a GI of 55 or less is considered low.

One problem with the glycemic index is that it detects only carbohydrate quality, not quantity. A GI value tells you only how rapidly a particular carbohydrate turns into sugar. It doesn't tell you how much of that carbohydrate is in a serving of a particular food. You need to know both things to understand a food's effect on blood sugar. The most famous example of this is the carrot. The form of sugar in the carrot has a high glycemic index, but the total carbohydrate content of the carrot is low, so it doesn't add a lot of calories. The term for this is glycemic load (GL), and it is calculated by taking the glycemic index, dividing it by 100, and multiplying it by its available carbohydrate content (i.e., carbohydrates minus fiber) in grams. A low GL is less than 16.

Glycemic load has been found to be the most important variable in studies of populations and their risk of chronic disease. So, populations eating a diet that has a high glycemic load, such as the U.S. diet of processed grains and few fruits and vegetables, have a higher risk of diabetes and heart disease than some Asian countries where lots of fruits and vegetables with few processed foods are eaten. This has been documented both in population studies, such as those conducted by the Harvard School of Public Health, and in weight-loss studies in children conducted at Children's Hospital in Boston, where a low GL diet was more effective in promoting weight loss than a high GL diet.

You are not going to be able to eat all low GL foods, but it is important to know both the GL and the calories that the food provides. One problem with GL is that some fatty foods that carry lots of calories can still have a lower glycemic index. The guides below are for your information in selecting or limiting carbohydrate-containing foods and some foods that falsely brag about their low glycemic index and load.

It is still true that every food has both a biochemistry side and a behavioral side. In these tables, I have put an asterisk on those foods most likely to be Trigger Foods, although any food can be a Trigger Food. (Even though a vegetable such as a cucumber has a low glycemic index, low glycemic load, and low calories, it is possible to gain weight by eating huge quantities of cucumbers. I actually had a patient who did this.)

If you want to lose weight, you are best off eating the low-calorie foods in the *low-GI, low-GL* or *high-GI, low-GL* categories. You want to stay away from the *high-GL, high-GI* group, and many of those are—not surprisingly—also Trigger Foods. However, you can't stop there. Even fatty foods that have a low glycemic index and glycemic load can have a lot of calories. Tree nuts have healthy oils, but I suggest you use them to add taste to a dish, or eat about eight nuts after a workout. Eating handfuls of salted nuts will put lots of calories in your body very quickly.

Glycemic Index, Glycemic Load, and Calories

The glycemic index, glycemic load, and total calories of various foods are listed in the table. Most of the GI values shown are based on 120 studies in the professional literature, referenced in the *American Journal of Clinical Nutrition,* July 2002. Foods with an asterisk are included in the Trigger Food list on page 34.

LOW-GI (<55) AND LOW-GL (<16) FOODS

Lowest Calorie (110 calories per serving or less)

	GI	GL	Serving Size	Calories
Most vegetables	<20	<5	1 cup, cooked	40
Apple	40	6	1 average	75
Banana	52	12	1 average	90
Cherries*	22	3	15 cherries	85
Grapefruit	25	5	1 average	75
Kiwi	53	6	1 average	45
Mango	51	14	1 small	110
Orange	48	5	1 average	65
Peach	42	7	1 average	70
Plums	39	5	2 medium	70
Strawberries	40	1	1 cup	50
Tomato juice	38	4	1 cup	40

HIGH-GI (>55) BUT LOW-GL (< 16) FOODS

All Low Calorie (110 or less)

	GI	GL	Serving Size	Calories
Apricots	57	6	4 medium	70
Orange juice*	57	15	1 cup	110
Papaya	60	9	1 cup cubes	55
Pineapple	59	7	1 cup cubes	75
Pumpkin	75	3	1 cup, mashed	85
Shredded wheat	75	15	1 cup mini squares	110
Watermelon	72	7	1 cup cubes	50

MODERATE CALORIE LOW GI, LOW GL

(110 to 135 calories per serving or less)

	GI	GL	Serving Size	Calories
Apple juice*	40	12	1 cup	135
Grapefruit juice*	48	9	1 cup	115
Pear	33	10	1 medium	125
Peas	48	3	1 cup	135
Pineapple juice*	46	15	1 cup	130
Whole-grain bread	51	14	1 slice	80–120

HIGHER CALORIE LOW GI, LOW GL

(160 to 300 calories per serving)

	GI	GL	Serving Size	Calories
Barley	25	11	1 cup, cooked	190
Black beans	20	8	1 cup, cooked	235
Garbanzo beans	28	13	1 cup, cooked	285
Grapes*	46	13	40 grapes	160
Kidney beans	23	10	1 cup, cooked	210
Lentils	29	7	1 cup, cooked	230
Soybeans	18	1	1 cup, cooked	300
Yam	37	13	1 cup, cooked	160

LOW GI AND LOW GL, BUT HIGH FAT AND HIGH CALORIE

	GI	GL	Serving Size	Calories
Cashews*	22	4	½ cup	395
Premium ice cream*	38	10	1 cup	360
Low-fat ice cream*	37–50	13	1 cup	220
Peanuts*	14	1	½ cup	330
Popcorn (full fat)	72	16	2 cups	110

	GI	GL	Serving Size	Calories
Potato chips*	54	15	2 ounces	345
Whole milk	27	3	1 cup	150
Vanilla pudding	44	16	1 cup	250
Fruit yogurt*	31	9	1 cup	200+
Soy yogurt	50	13	1 cup	200+

HIGH GI ≥ 55 HIGH GL ≥ 16

Many Trigger Foods, Many Higher Calorie

	GI	GL	Serving Size	Calories
Baked potato	85	34	1 small	220
Brown rice	55	16	1 cup	215
Cola*	63	33	16-ounce bottle	200
Corn	60	20	1 ear, 1 cup kernels	130
Corn chips*	63	21	2 ounces	350
Corn flakes	92	24	1 cup	100
Cream of wheat	74	22	1 cup, cooked	130
Croissant*	67	17	1 average	275
French fries*	75	25	1 large order	515
Macaroni & cheese*	64	46	1 cup	285
Pizza*	60	20	1 large slice	300
Pretzels*	83	33	1 ounce	115
Raisin Bran	61	29	1 cup	185
Raisins	66	42	½ cup	250
Soda crackers*	74	18	12 crackers	155
Waffles	76	18	1 average	150
White bread*	73	20	2 small slices	160
White rice*	64	23	1 cup, cooked	210

It's Not the Fish, It's the Aquarium

Rather than blame the dieter, I like to say, "It's not the fish, it's the aquarium." How can you be expected to lose weight when you are surrounded by the wrong triggers and the wrong foods? In this chapter you have learned how to build your personal best diet to achieve your personal-best shape. This is not a "one size fits all" diet plan, as you can see, but the most up-to-date understanding of foods that science has today. However, food is not the whole story. You will need to transform your life to eliminate as much as possible the constant stress, inactivity, and overeating that has you trapped, and to build a life that is fulfilling and healthy, balancing your physical activity and new eating habits with time for relaxation and reflection.

One thing that has helped my patients to evaluate their eating habits is maintaining a food diary (you'll find a sample in the Appendix). First, you need to set your daily goals, and then you can transfer them to your own diary or calendar. Use the following checklist to plan out what you will be recording in your diary. I recommend looking at a week at a time so that you can observe your dietary patterns. Then you can come back to this chapter and see if there is more you can do to reach your goals. Now that you know what to do, here is your Personal Checklist for designing your ideal personalized diet:

Personal Diet Checklist/Daily Goals

Date:

Protein : Total Gram Target _____ grams = _____ 25-gm units

    Breakfast _____

    Lunch _____

    P.M. Snack _____

    Dinner _____

Fruits and Vegetables Target = 7 servings (one from each color)

    Breakfast _____

    Lunch _____

    P.M. Snack _____

    Dinner _____

Fiber Target = 25 Grams = 5 units of 5 grams or more

    Breakfast _____

    Lunch _____

    P.M. Snack _____

    Dinner _____

Grain Servings 1–3 Servings: Fiber _____ Calories _____

Remember to add up the totals for each category you have listed above and check to see that you attained your personal targets for grams of protein, seven servings of fruits and vegetables, and 25 grams of fiber per day for a typical day. Obviously, you won't eat the same way every day, but this exercise can be repeated and will serve as a reality check to see that you are close to your targets. You can use a computer or personal digital assistant (PDA) to record your food intake. In my experience, most people don't want to go to all the trouble of recording food intake every day, but it is a good idea to do it for at least a few days in order to see that you are hitting your personal targets.

The Next Step

Now that you have set your goals, Step 3 will show you how to activate your personal plan, with menu plans, shopping lists, simple recipes, travel tips, and holiday eating plans.

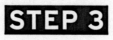
STEP 3

Activating Your
Personal Plan

Once you have passed the first week of weight loss, you have reached an important milestone. You have learned that you can lose weight, and you have made that very important first step of committing to a lifestyle change.

Over the next week you will learn how to change your diet in simple ways that will help you manage your weight for a lifetime. After powering through the first week with two shakes per day, you can and should consider still using meal replacements twice a day to boost your weight loss efforts until you reach your target. One meal replacement a day will keep you progressing toward your target weight, but at a slower rate.

However, this book is not just about losing weight but rather about preparing you to keep your healthy weight once you reach your target. You can begin practicing with one meal a day as you continue to lose weight and avoiding, cutting down, or controlling your Trigger Foods. This process goes on for a long time, not just the twelve weeks promised in some books. Research by my colleagues demonstrates that meal replacement is a strategy that improves your ability to stick with a healthy diet over the long term.

Here is what you will learn:

- How to plan your daily menu and organize your shopping

- How to replace foods that have hidden vegetable oils and added re-fined sugar with healthy, great-tasting foods that are high in fiber and satisfy your hunger with protein and fiber

- How to control the environment in restaurants when you eat away from home so that you get adequate protein at each meal to maintain your muscles

- How not to be hungry without going on an unhealthy high-fat, high-protein diet

- How to prepare to maintain your plan while traveling

- How to reorganize your pantry, because you can't eat foods you don't buy or bring into your house

- Simple, quick recipes to put your personal plan into action

- Terrific recipes for special occasions

- How to survive holiday eating without losing control of your plan

- How to avoid some of the most common food and dieting myths out there that can steer you away from your plan

Planning Your Menu and Shopping

If you lived in the wild, your problem every day would be finding enough food to eat. Today, existing hunter-gatherer populations are very knowledge-able about the plants in their local area. They know which ones are healthy to eat and which ones need to be cooked first to be safe to eat. They have learned how to do some primitive farming to keep a supply of some staple foods, usually starches. They understand that variety is needed, because sickness follows when the diet becomes dependent on only one of these crop foods.

What does this have to do with modern-day America? The fact is that most Americans are not getting the nutrition they need from their foods. They settle into monotonous diets with too many brown-beige foods and not enough fruits and vegetables. Today our selection of foods is determined by taste, cost, and convenience, rather than by the careful selection process that humans evolved over millions of years in the wild. So, you need a plan to help you select a healthy diet.

When you enter the grocery store, start in the produce section, not the packaged-goods section. There are some healthy foods in the packaged-goods, dairy, and meat sections, but you should first select fruits and vegetables, which have the lowest numbers of calories per bite. We all know that fruits and vegetables are healthy, but you need to strictly limit or avoid fruit juices, dried fruits, nuts, and most starchy vegetables, such as beans and potatoes. It takes more than two oranges to make a glass of orange juice. I would rather that you ate the whole orange.

Look for the best sources of protein, including lean meats, chicken, and fish, or the new soy meat substitutes. While beans and rice and nuts are major sources of protein in many underdeveloped countries around the world, rice and beans have about 250 calories per cup, and a cup of nuts can have as many as 800 calories. However, populations in underdeveloped countries are usually much more active than we are and need the calories these foods provide to maintain their high levels of physical activity. When individuals immigrate from those countries to the U.S. and continue to eat rice and beans while adding high-calorie meats to their diet, they quickly begin to gain weight. This is also happening in the urban areas of many of these developing countries, contributing to the worldwide epidemic of obesity. So you will be learning to cut back on beans, rice, pasta, potatoes, and crackers.

I am not too proud to change my message when the science changes. Just ten years ago, I would have told you that a diet rich in pasta is healthy because it is low fat. Now we know that in terms of gaining weight, eating refined sugars and starches can cause you to lose control of your diet, especially if you are a carbohydrate craver.

Week Two : Menus for Changing Your Shape

Before you start shopping, you need to know what you plan to eat. Here are a week's worth of menus for men and women, followed by a shopping list that provides not only the ingredients you need to prepare the recipes, but a list of foods you should keep in your pantry, refrigerator, and freezer.

Once your pantry and refrigerator are stocked with healthy foods and you have cleared out the high-calorie items, it's not a struggle to prepare a quick, healthy meal. If you are on the meal replacement plan, just use one of two of the meal suggestions per day and shop accordingly.

Try your best to get seven or more servings of fruits and vegetables of different colors into your diet each day, and you will be doing far better than 80 percent of all Americans in terms of fruit and vegetable intake. You will be keeping your weight loss going, since most fruits and vegetables are low in calories per bite so you can eat more and weigh less.

The National Cancer Institute recommends five to nine servings per day, with nine for men and five for children. Women and teenagers should have seven servings. Countries with lower rates of cancer and heart disease than the United States eat more than a pound of fruits and vegetables a day, which is about seven to nine servings. You will notice in the menu plans that the color group of fruits and vegetables as outlined in the last chapter is included for your use in eating a diverse selection.

A Week's Menus—Women

You can personalize the amounts of protein according to your lean body mass, with some men needing 35 grams and some women needing only 20 grams. Whatever your personal protein level turns out to be, you will find that your hunger is satisfied as never before.

Day One

Breakfast: Blueberry or strawberry soy protein shake with additional protein added to reach your personal protein prescription

    Place in blender:

    Soy protein powder

    Protein powder as needed for your personal protein target

    With 1 cup soy milk or 1 cup nonfat milk

    + 1 cup fresh or frozen blueberries or strawberries (*red/purple*)

    + A few ice cubes

Lunch: *(Note: Drink another soy protein shake on the two-meal replacement plan, or eat this lunch and a meal replacement for dinner,*

Recipes marked* begin on page 102.

or eat a regular lunch and dinner for slower weight loss. The choice is yours, but stick with what you pick for this week. Later on, you can use any plan you want on a given day.)

> Seafood salad made with:
> Chunk light water-packed tuna
> Imitation crabmeat
> Tomatoes (*red*)
> Celery, parsley, and green onion (*white/green*)
> Served on a bed of romaine lettuce (*yellow/green*)
> Dressed with *L.A. Shape "Green Goddess" Dressing (*yellow/green*)

Snack: One 6- to 8-inch banana, or 1 whole orange, sliced (*yellow/orange*)

Dinner: *Chicken and Turkey Meat Loaf
           Steamed broccoli (*green*) and carrots (*orange*)
           Baked apple with cinnamon (*red/purple*)

Day Two

Breakfast: Soy shake as on Day One (or any shake recipe from Week One) or:
           Soy cereal with fruit
           ½ cup soy nugget cereal (see Appendix)
           1 cup nonfat milk
           1 cup fresh berries (*red/purple*)

Lunch: Any soy shake, or:
           Chicken and fruit salad made with:
           Roasted chicken breast, shredded

Diced celery (*white/green*)

Cucumber (*white/green*)

Red apple, diced (*red/purple*)

Carrot (*orange*)

Bed of romaine lettuce (*yellow/green*)

Tossed with *L.A. Shape Carrot Vinaigrette (*orange*)

Snack: 1 whole orange (*orange/yellow*)

Dinner: *Gazpacho (*red*)

Grilled fresh fish: snapper, sole, or halibut

Sautéed spinach (*yellow/green*) with scallions (*white/green*)

Fresh fruit

Day Three

Breakfast: Soy shake as on Day One (or any shake recipe from Week One), or:

7 egg whites or 1 cup Egg Beaters, scrambled with onion, chives, and fresh herbs (*white/green*)

1 slice high-fiber whole wheat bread (70 to 100 calories and 5 to 7 grams of fiber), toasted

Sliced cantaloupe or other melon (*yellow/orange*)

Lunch: Any soy shake, or:

Turkey/avocado chopped vegetable salad made with:

Roasted turkey breast

Avocado (*yellow/green*)

Tomato (*red*)

Broccoli (*green*)

Cucumber (*white/green*)

Carrot (*orange*)

Red bell pepper (*red*)

Yellow bell pepper (*yellow/orange*)

Tossed with *L.A. Shape Orange-Ginger Dressing (*orange/yellow*)

Snack: 1 cup fresh or frozen blackberries or blueberries (*red/purple*)

Dinner: *Soy chili

Salad of mixed field greens with *L.A. Shape "Green Goddess" Dressing (*yellow/green*)

1 fresh red apple (*red/purple*)

Day Four

Breakfast: Soy shake as on Day One (or any shake recipe from Week One), or:

1 cup nonfat cottage cheese, sprinkled with cinnamon

1 slice high-fiber/low calorie whole-grain bread, toasted

3 slices soy Canadian bacon

1 cup diced pineapple (*orange/yellow*)

Lunch: Any soy shake, or:

Mixed vegetable salad topped with chicken soy patty and any *L.A. Shape Dressing

Snack: 1½ cups fresh strawberries (*red/purple*)

Dinner: *Roasted Eggplant Salad (*red/purple; red; white/green*)

Shrimp or fish and vegetable skewers seasoned with lemon and oregano

1 whole orange (*orange/yellow*)

Day Five

Breakfast:	Soy shake as on Day One (or any shake recipe from Week One), or:

Breakfast burrito:

    2 corn tortillas, filled with:

    4 scrambled egg whites

    1 soy sausage patty, cooked and crumbled

    ⅛ avocado (*yellow/green*)

    Fresh tomato salsa (*red*)

    1½ large papaya with lime juice (*orange/yellow*)

Lunch: Any soy shake, or:

Chicken vegetable bowl:

One grilled chicken breast on top of

Steamed broccoli (*green*)

Chinese cabbage (*green*)

Steamed carrots (*orange*)

Topped with bottled teriyaki sauce

Snack: 1½ cups mixed berries (*red/purple*)

Dinner: *Indian Chicken Curry with

*Cucumber and Yogurt Salad (*white/green*)

1 large kiwi, diced (*yellow/green*) with a handful of raspberries (*red/purple*)

Day Six

Breakfast: Soy shake as on Day One, or:

Egg white omelet with herbs:

7 egg whites made into an omelet and filled with:

The L.A. Shape Diet

Fresh mushrooms (*white/green*)

Fresh thyme, rosemary, herbs of choice

1 slice whole-grain bread

½ medium cantaloupe (*orange/yellow*)

Lunch: Any soy shake, or:

*Quick California Rolls

Cherry tomato salad with *L.A. Shape Dressing (*red*)

Snack: One 6- to 8-inch banana

Dinner: *Creamy Butternut Squash Soup (*orange*)

*Sherry-Braised Chicken and Mushrooms

Steamed mixed vegetables

1 cup strawberries (*red/purple*)

Day Seven

Breakfast: Soy shake or any shake recipe from Week One

Fresh fruit and yogurt/soy sundae:

Fruit salad of berries, peaches, and pineapple (*red/purple;
orange/yellow*) on top of:

1 cup plain yogurt mixed with

2 tablespoons soy protein powder (10 grams)

Sprinkle with cinnamon, a drizzle of honey, and soy cereal
for crunch

1 slice whole-grain toast

Lunch: Any soy shake, or:

Chef's salad:

Romaine lettuce and spinach leaves (*yellow/green*)

Activating Your Personal Plan

Green onion (*white/green*)

Tomato (*red*)

Hard-boiled egg whites and vegetarian turkey

Tossed with any *L.A. Shape Dressing

Snack: Deep dark chocolate soy protein pudding:

1 tablespoon chocolate soy protein powder (5 grams of
protein)

½ cup soy milk

Blend in 1 tablespoon fat-free cocoa powder

Refrigerate for 20 minutes and top with ½ teaspoon
powdered sugar

Dinner: *Thai-Style Scallops

Sautéed baby bok choy, onions, and garlic (*green;
white/green*)

1 whole orange (*orange*)

A Week's Menus—Men

Day One

Breakfast: Blueberry or strawberry soy protein shake (or any shake
recipe from Week One) and added protein powder to reach
your personal protein target.

Place in blender:

Soy protein powder with 1 cup soy milk or 1 cup nonfat
milk

Added protein powder

+ 1 cup fresh or frozen blueberries or strawberries (*red/purple*)

+ A few ice cubes

1 cup of coffee or green or black tea

Lunch:	Any soy shake or:
	Seafood salad made with:
	Chunk light water-packed tuna
	Imitation crabmeat
	Tomatoes (*red*)
	Celery, parsley, and green onion (*white/green*)
	Served on a bed of romaine lettuce (*yellow/green*)
	Dressed with *L.A. Shape "Green Goddess" Dressing (*yellow/green*)
	1 slice 100 percent whole-grain bread
Snack:	High-protein bar and an apple or banana
Dinner:	*Chicken and Turkey Meat Loaf
	Broccoli (*green*) and carrots (*orange*) steamed with garlic
	½ cup brown rice
	Baked apple with cinnamon (*red/purple*)

Day Two

Breakfast:	Soy shake as on Day One (or any shake recipe from Week One) fortified with additional protein powder to meet your personal protein target.
	½ grapefruit or whole orange, not juice (*orange/yellow*)

Lunch:	Chicken and fruit salad made with:
	Two roasted chicken breasts (50 gm protein), shredded
	Diced celery (*white/green*)
	Cucumber (*white/green*)
	Red apple, diced(*red/purple*)
	Carrot (*orange*)
	Tossed with *L.A. Shape Carrot Vinaigrette (*orange*)
	Placed on a bed of romaine lettuce (*yellow/green*)
	1 slice 100 percent whole-grain bread

Snack:	2 ounces soy nuts and 1 orange

Dinner:	*Gazpacho (*red*)
	Grilled fresh fish
	Sautéed spinach and scallions (*yellow/green; white/green*)
	1 ear corn on the cob (*yellow/green*)
	½ fresh mango or papaya with lime juice (*orange*)

Day Three

Breakfast:	Soy shake as on Day One (or any shake recipe from Week One) fortified with additional protein powder to meet your personal protein target.
	Or:
	Egg breakfast:
	7 egg whites, scrambled with onion, chives, and fresh herbs (*white/green*)
	1 cup frozen or fresh mixed vegetables or spinach, sautéed (*yellow /green*)
	1 or 2 slices high-fiber whole-grain bread, toasted
	Coffee or green or black tea (optional)

Lunch:	Any soy shake, or:

Lunch:

Any soy shake, or:

Turkey/avocado chopped vegetable salad made with:

6 ounces roasted turkey breast

½ fresh avocado (*yellow/green*)

1 sliced tomato (*red*)

Broccoli (*green*)

Cucumber (*white/green*)

Carrot (*orange*)

Red bell pepper (*red*)

Yellow bell pepper (*yellow/orange*)

Toss with *L.A. Shape Orange-Ginger Dressing (*yellow/orange*)

1 slice whole-grain bread

Cantaloupe and honeydew melon chunks (*yellow/orange*)

Green tea or coffee (optional)

Snack:

Quick soy fruit pudding

Blend in a blender:

2 to 3 tablespoons vanilla soy-protein powder (15 gm protein)

¼ cup nonfat soy milk or nonfat milk

1 cup fresh or frozen mixed berries (*red/purple*)

Refrigerate or let set as pudding

Dinner:

*Soy chili with ½ cup beans added

Salad of mixed field greens with any *L.A. Shape Dressing

1 fresh red apple (*red/purple*)

Day Four

Breakfast:	Soy shake as on Day One (or any shake recipe from Week One) fortified with additional protein powder to meet your personal protein target

Or:

Cottage cheese, soy burger, and fruit breakfast:

1 cup nonfat cottage cheese (25 gm protein)

1 soy burger patty, grilled

1 cup fresh blackberries and raspberries (*red/purple*)

Lunch:	Any soy shake, or:

Mixed vegetable salad topped with chicken soy patty

Any *L.A. Shape Dressing

1 slice whole-grain bread

Melon or strawberries

Coffee or green tea (optional)

Snack:	1 ounce roasted soy nuts and a piece of fruit (apple or pear)

Dinner:	*Roasted Eggplant Salad (*red/purple; red; white/green*)

Shrimp or fish and vegetable skewers seasoned with lemon and oregano

½ 100 percent whole-grain pita bread

1 whole orange (*orange/yellow*)

Day Five

Breakfast:	Soy shake as on Day One (or any shake recipe from Week One) fortified with additional protein powder to meet your personal protein target.

Or:

South of the Border Burrito Breakfast:

    Two corn tortillas, filled with:

    7 egg whites, scrambled (25 gm protein)

    2 soy sausages (25 gm protein)

    ½ avocado (*yellow/green*)

    Fresh tomato salsa (*red*)

    ½ large papaya garnished with lime juice (*orange/ yellow*)

Lunch: Any soy shake, or:

Chicken and vegetable bowl:

Two grilled chicken breasts (50 gm protein)

Broccoli (*green*)

Chinese cabbage (*green*)

Steamed carrots (*orange*)

Topped with bottled teriyaki sauce

½ cup steamed brown rice

½ cantaloupe or honeydew melon (*orange/yellow; yellow/green*)

Snack: Protein bar (25 gm protein)

Dinner: *Indian Chicken Curry with

*Cucumber and Yogurt Salad (*white/green*)

½ cup cooked garbanzo beans or lentils added to curry

Large kiwi, diced (*yellow/green*): with 1 cup raspberries (*red/purple*)

Day Six

Breakfast: Soy shake as on Day One (or any shake recipe from Week One) fortified with additional protein powder to meet your personal protein target or:

Egg white omelet with herbs:

7 egg-white omelet (25 gm protein), filled with:

Fresh mushrooms (*white/green*)

Fresh thyme, rosemary, or other herbs of choice

Soy Canadian bacon (25 gm)

1 slice whole-grain bread, toasted

½ medium cantaloupe (*orange/yellow*)

Lunch: Any soy shake, or:

*Quick California Rolls

½ cup steamed brown rice

Cherry tomato salad with any *L.A. Shape Dressing (*red*)

Snack: 1 cup vegetarian chili

Dinner: *Creamy Butternut Squash Soup (*orange*)

*Wine-Braised Chicken Strips

Steamed mixed vegetables

One 100 percent whole-grain dinner roll

1 cup strawberries (*red/purple*)

Day Seven

Breakfast: Soy shake as on Day One (or any shake recipe from Week One) fortified with additional protein powder to meet your personal protein target, or:

Fresh fruit and yogurt soy sundae with soy patty.

Fruit salad of berries, peaches, and pineapple (*red/purple; orange/yellow*) on top of:

1 cup plain yogurt (14 gm protein)

Sprinkle with ¼ cup high-protein soy cereal for crunch (5 gm protein)

Soy meat substitute patty, grilled (25 gm protein)

1 slice whole-grain toast

Coffee or green tea (optional)

Lunch: Any soy shake, or:

Chef's turkey salad:

6 ounces sliced smoked turkey breast (50 gm protein)

Romaine lettuce and spinach leaves (*yellow/green*)

Tomato (*red*)

Tossed with any *L.A. Shape Dressing

1 slice whole-grain high-fiber wheat bread

Snack: High-protein bar and a fruit

Dinner: *Thai-Style Scallops

Sautéed baby bok choy with garlic (*green; white/green*)

½ cup steamed brown rice

1 orange (*orange/yellow*)

Shopping Guidelines

You don't need to shop every day, but you do want your foods to be as fresh as possible. Most of the foods on these lists will keep for a few days, with the exception of fresh fish. If you prefer fresh fish over frozen, you will

Activating Your Personal Plan

need to make a special stop for fresh fish, since it should be eaten within twenty-four hours of buying it. The supplies listed below will enable you to prepare the meals outlined above, and will help you to get your pantry stocked with healthy items.

SHOPPING LIST

√ Meat/Fish/Poultry

Canned, water-packed light or albacore tuna

Chicken breasts, fresh or frozen

Canned water-packed chicken breast or turkey breast

Fresh or frozen fish and scallops

Imitation crabmeat

Shrimp, fresh or frozen

Turkey breast half for roasting

√ Soy Protein

Frozen soy burger or soy chicken patties

Soft tofu

High-protein bars

Plain soy milk

Roasted soy nuts

Soy Canadian bacon

Soy "ground round"

Soy protein isolate powder, plain and flavored

Soy sausage patties

Vegetarian turkey slices

√ Fruits

Apples, fresh and frozen slices

Bananas

Berries, fresh or frozen

Cantaloupe

Cranberry juice, low-calorie

Kiwi

Lemons

Limes

Mandarin oranges, canned

Mango, fresh or frozen chunks

Papaya

Peaches, fresh and frozen slices

Pineapple

Orange juice concentrate

Oranges

√ Vegetables

Avocado

Baby-food carrots and green beans

Beans, pinto, garbanzo, or black, canned

Broccoli

Butternut squash, frozen

Cabbage, green, red, Chinese, and/or purple

Carrots

Celery

Chilis, green, canned

Cilantro

Corn, fresh or frozen

Cucumber

Eggplant

Garlic

Ginger, fresh

Green beans, fresh or frozen

Mixed leafy greens

Mixed vegetables, frozen

Mushrooms

Onions, red and yellow

Parsley

Peppers, green, yellow and red, fresh or frozen

Pumpkin, canned

Romaine lettuce

Scallions

Spinach, fresh

Tomatoes, whole, cherry, canned

Tomato juice

Tomato sauce

Water chestnuts, canned

Zucchini

√ *Dairy*

Egg whites and egg substitutes

Cottage cheese, nonfat

Dry milk, nonfat

Milk, nonfat or skim

Yogurt, plain nonfat

√ Grains

Brown rice

Corn tortillas

100 percent whole-grain bread

100 percent whole-grain dinner rolls

100 percent whole-grain pita bread

√ Seasonings

Chicken bouillon granules

Dried herbs and spices

Extracts, vanilla, orange, lemon, black walnut, coconut

Hot red pepper flakes

Lemon chicken sauce mix

Tabasco sauce

Unsweetened cocoa powder

√ Miscellaneous

Barbecue sauce

Bread crumbs

Broth, canned: chicken or vegetable

Hoisin sauce

Honey

Ketchup

Mustard, yellow and Dijon

Olive oil

Oyster-flavored sauce

Soy sauce

Steak sauce

Sweet-and-sour sauce

Tea bags

Tea concentrate, liquid, unsweetened

Teriyaki sauce

Thai fish sauce

Tomato salsa

Vinegars, balsamic, rice, wine, tarragon

Worcestershire sauce

Olive oil spray

Dining Out

It may seem simple, but looking at your food before you eat it is the first step in controlling your food habits. Some foods, such as the inside of a burger bun, are usually hidden from view. Did you know that restaurants smear the inside of your refined-grain bun with mayonnaise before they add iceberg lettuce and ketchup to your high-fat burger? This is no joke. In just twenty years, we have gone from a small 280-calorie burger with a pickle and ketchup to a double cheeseburger with 1,280 calories. Open up the bun and look at the melted cheese, mayonnaise, or Thousand Island dressing and the fatty meat patty.

You can do something about it the next time you are faced with having to eat a fast-food meal because you are trapped in an airport. If they have it, order the grilled chicken sandwich with no mayo. *Always hold the mayo.* Mayonnaise is simply lots of vegetable oil with whole eggs mixed in a blender. It is added to affect mouth feel. Artificial flavors made from chemicals extracted from beef hides are also used in the burger and fries.

Now let's go to a better restaurant. You are about to be served dinner. The choices are prime rib, chicken, halibut, and farmed salmon. They are served with rice pilaf or mashed potatoes and a salad that comes with Thousand Island or ranch dressing. Dessert is either chocolate cake, ice cream, sherbet, or mixed fruit. Have you decided? If you picked the prime rib and mashed potatoes, add 1,750 calories to your day's intake. If you picked the ranch dressing on your salad, add another 100 calories. You're up to 1,850. Now add 350 calories for ice cream or chocolate cake, and you have eaten 2,100 calories in one meal. Even with exercise, this is 500 calories more than most women need for the whole day.

Now, let's turn back the clock, and the waiter appears again. Pick the breast of chicken with no skin or the halibut, and have them grilled to perfection. Ask for a double serving of mixed steamed vegetables, including broccoli and carrots, dress your salad with a nice balsamic vinegar, and have the mixed fruit for dessert. Sounds pretty good—and there are 300 calories in the fish or chicken, 80 in the mixed vegetables, 30 in the salad, and 70 in the dessert, for a total of 480 calories.

You're on the right track—until the waiter's a little slow and you start digging around in the bread basket. Three pieces of bread give you an additional 300 calories! The most grains you need in a day are two or three slices of high-fiber bread and a bowl of high-fiber cereal. I am not a sugar buster or fat buster, but I am against unconsciously letting your calories run up because you don't look at what you are putting into your mouth. Ask the waiter to bring you some cut-up vegetables to chew on while you wait, or simply ask for the salad right away with some water and lemon.

Now, how about some wine or beer? Wine is the better choice. Beer is a refined grain, with 220 calories in a regular beer and about 300 in that giant 24-ounce mug. Wine is about 90 calories a glass, and the red wines contain healthy phytochemicals. So here you can save another 130 to 210 calories—and it all adds up. Wine consumed responsibly is also a stress re-

Tips For Dining Out

1. If there are chips or bread on the table when you sit down, move them as far away from you as possible. A single serving of high-fat tortilla chips fried in oil is over 500 calories, and those wonderful breads and rolls add up quickly to hundreds of calories. If your waiter or waitress tries to serve bread or chips, ask that he or she take your order and remove the chips or bread. At some restaurants they offer cut-up vegetables (crudités). Ask for veggies instead of bread if you are really hungry, or have a glass of water or iced tea and make some good conversation until your food arrives.

2. Order a salad with dark greens—not iceberg lettuce—with wine, rice, or balsamic vinegar. Have as many things added to the salad as possible that provide taste without lots of extra calories, such as red peppers, green peppers, carrots, broccoli, or alfalfa sprouts. You can have a big salad— just pass up the fat-filled dressings.

3. Order a meat entrée that is low in fat, such as chicken breast, white meat of turkey, white fish, seafood, or lean meat cuts. Use the chart on protein units on pages 50–51 to see how many ounces you need to eat.

4. Select at least two different colors of vegetables and make sure the size of the vegetable serving is at least twice the size of your protein serving.

5. For dessert, order a bowl of mixed fruits, such as strawberries, raspberries, and kiwi fruit. If they're not available, ask for an orange, apple, or pear on a plate. Some restaurants offer a baked apple or pear seasoned with cinnamon. Be sure they don't drown them in sugary syrup, and then enjoy. Cut any of these fresh or baked fruit desserts up with a fork and knife and eat them slowly, savoring the flavor as if you were eating a high-fat/high-sugar cake, pastry, or pie.

ducer and can make even the most provincial meal seem special. If you absolutely prefer beer, have a light beer (110 calories). Of course, if you have a problem with alcohol, ignore what I just wrote.

Don't fall into the "more is better" trap! Since most restaurant costs relate to labor, they think they can get you to come back by serving you lots of food at a low price. If you are offered an entrée with a starch and vegetables, ask for no starch and double the vegetables, and add a vegetable soup or salad to your meal.

The exception to this rule is the class of high-priced restaurants where presentation is more important than quantity. These restaurants use multicolored sauces to surround small portions of meat, fish, or poultry surrounded by beautifully treated, but sometimes skimpy, amounts of vegetables. However, it is usually easy to ask for more steamed vegetables or to order a separate vegetable dish. Continental cooks know the value of multicolored dining.

Restaurant dining should be a pleasurable experience that focuses on much more than just the food. When you walk into a restaurant, visualize sitting down to a fine social experience. It used to be that we only ate out on special occasions such as birthdays or anniversaries. Today Americans eat out at least 50 percent of the time.

Often we eat out during the week, because there's no time to cook. There might be a special event for your kids, a PTA meeting or athletic event, or you might just have a business meeting that ran late. When you find you are eating out during the week, don't reward yourself for a hard day's work with a huge meal, or think that you can bury your anxiety by filling your stomach with high-fat foods, such as steak and onion rings. You are not a lumberjack, and you shouldn't eat like one. If you need to chomp on something, start your meal with a large salad with wine vinegar or lemon followed by a big plate of steamed vegetables or a vegetable soup. By concentrating on getting your fruits, vegetables, and protein first, you will be eating more food with fewer calories than most foods you can find on a restaurant menu.

Controlling the amount of fat you eat is another huge hurdle in restaurants, because fats can be found everywhere: on the table (butter, margarine, chips), in meal preparation (fried, smothered), and in the ingredients themselves (butter, cheese). Since you aren't preparing the food, learn to ask the right questions about ingredients and preparation so that you can get what you want.

- Ask that fish or chicken be baked or broiled, not deep-fried.

- Ask for sauces on the side or ask to have butter or cream sauces left out altogether.

- Ask to substitute a double serving of steamed vegetables without butter or sauce for rice or potatoes.

Waiters in some restaurants dominate the agenda as they recite mouthwatering specials on the menu. Don't be intimidated. It's not rude to ask how a food is prepared! After all, you are the customer. While you can't reasonably ask for something that isn't even remotely like any item on the menu, you *can* ask for modified dishes—by omitting certain ingredients, or having dressings and sauces omitted or served on the side.

Get familiar with cooking terms: Lower-fat items are roasted, poached, steamed, grilled, broiled, or stir-fried, but crispy, creamy, breaded, scalloped, or au gratin foods are high in fat. Vinaigrette salad dressings contain both oil and vinegar—have them served on the side, not tossed, so you can control the amount you eat.

Read the entire menu, too. Vegetables may not be abundant when served with an entrée, but check the salads, side dishes, and appetizer sections on the menu to supplement your meals and to help meet your fruit and vegetable goals. You are in charge. The restaurant business is tough, and they need you more than you need them.

Eating at Home

If you are eating dinner at home, how can you fix something in under fifteen minutes so you don't have to order a pizza? You can grill chicken breasts, fish fillets, or soy burgers. There are many electric grills that will drain off the excess fat and give you great grilled flavor. Now, take frozen vegetables from a big freezer bag, throw them in a dish, and steam them in the microwave. Top with the grilled meat and some barbecue, soy, or teriyaki sauce, and you have just saved yourself money and time. Packaged salads are already cut up and washed, and you can add a rice vinegar, wine vinegar, or one of the low-fat L.A. Shape dressings to the salad. Dessert is simply fruit. While this is not difficult, it takes some planning.

Sadly, the modern American lifestyle offers us precious little time to slow down and enjoy healthy meals. By stocking your cupboard and refrigerator at home, you'll have easy access to foods that will help your health rather than simply adding to your waistline.

Traveling

It is possible (but not always easy) to stay with your *L.A. Shape* plan when traveling, but paying attention to diet and exercise while you are away from home makes the inevitable slips less damaging. On airplanes, avoid alcohol and snack chips or nuts. Instead ask for mixed vegetable or tomato juice, tea, or water. I usually pack a protein meal bar in my carry-on bag so that when the mystery meat arrives, I won't be without an alternative. Even when airline food is decent, I remove all the high-fat items from the plate and put them inside the plastic container that comes with the plastic fork and knife. Most airline meals in coach cost the airlines about $3.00, so you know the quality and freshness of the foods is not likely to be high.

If you arrive at your destination very late or very early in the day, you may find that most stores are closed. Again, the piece of fruit and the protein bar you packed will come in handy. In the morning, most hotels offer a breakfast buffet with fruits to start your day. Go for strawberries, honeydew melon, watermelon, and cantaloupe. If you are in a hotel or motel for several days with no breakfast buffet, keep some fruits and vegetables in a refrigerator in your room. Baby carrots, broccoli, cherry tomatoes, and some berries will tide you over for several days. Buy a few cans of mixed tomato–based vegetable juices in regular or spicy flavors. You can also keep some low-fat meats or soy meat substitutes in the refrigerator.

When you are away on business, you may go to some of the kinds of noteworthy restaurants you don't generally visit at home. Make it a habit to order the specialty of the house with the intention of tasting it and sharing it around your table. Make sure your entrée, salad, and vegetables conform to your *L.A. Shape* plan. While some deviations from the plan work, business trip meals filled with prime rib, creamed spinach, and mashed potatoes, accompanied by salted peanuts and Scotch, will just not fill the bill. While you may have good intentions of making up for your eating when you get home, the next business trip may be just around the corner.

Holiday Eating

Holidays can be full of stress. Traveling becomes more difficult, streets are crowded with shoppers, traffic slows, and your least favorite relatives show up at your house. Here are some key tips for keeping up your *L.A. Shape* plan during the holidays.

HOLIDAY OFFICE PARTIES

Get through these obligatory parties by having a glass of sparkling water with lime in it on ice. Then find a talkative person at the periphery of the party and keep your distance from the table with balls of cheese and nuts to tempt you off your plan. If you drink, try having a good-tasting red wine rather than hard liquor, and always have some protein, such as shrimp, fish, or chicken, with the alcohol to protect your stomach and balance your nutrition between protein and carbohydrate. Alcohol can inhibit your body's ability to keep up your blood sugar between meals, and I have seen people faint by having two drinks several hours after skipping their last meal. If you are involved in planning the party, make sure to have cut-up green and red peppers (holiday colors after all) and other colorful vegetables and fruits available at the party.

JULY FOURTH, MEMORIAL DAY, AND LABOR DAY

The traditional hot dog covered with mustard and relish can be replaced by a soy hot dog and the traditional burgers replaced with soy burgers. You'll be surprised at how closely they resemble the real thing, and you don't have to worry about what's in them. Grill shrimp, chicken breast pieces, or fish on skewers separated by onions, peppers, and other vegetables. Skewer two to four vegetables per piece of meat, fish, or seafood.

Activating Your Personal Plan

VALENTINE'S DAY, MOTHER'S DAY, AND FATHER'S DAY

Avoid the crush at restaurants and plan a healthy picnic or meal at home using the skills you have learned. Center your day around some special activity other than eating. Use the money you save to go to a movie or play or buy a thought-provoking book for your loved one.

Now we'll move on to the recipes—and the next chapter will help you reinforce your new behaviors.

Recipes

A WORD ABOUT THE SHAKE RECIPES

Since different brands of soy protein powders have varying amounts of flavorings and sweeteners, the recipes simply indicate a flavor such as vanilla or chocolate and the words "soy protein powder." You may need to adjust these recipes to suit your protein needs. Generally speaking, you should look for a shake mix that provides at least 9 grams of protein before you add your "mixer," which will usually be plain soy milk or nonfat milk. To this mixture you then add pure protein powder (usually 5 grams per tablespoon) to reach your personal protein target for that meal. While I prefer soy milk, this choice is not always available. Some people prefer nonfat milk—it's a high-quality animal protein, and your overall protein balance will still be just fine. A vanilla soy protein shake mix with added nonfat milk or plain soy milk makes a great base because the combination carries the added flavors so well. You'll notice that many recipes begin with these ingredients. Some plain (unflavored, unsweetened) soy powders have more protein per serving, but are more difficult to flavor properly. They taste best when mixed with fruit juices, but this can boost the calorie content too high. Start with the following recipes, which use either chocolate- or vanilla-flavored soy protein powder as the base.

PUMPKIN-BANANA SMOOTHIE

> 1 serving vanilla-flavored soy protein powder
> 1 cup plain soy milk or nonfat milk
> $1/4$ cup canned pumpkin (not pumpkin pie mix)
> $1/2$ medium banana
> A few drops vanilla extract
> Scant $1/8$ teaspoon pumpkin pie spice
> 4 ice cubes

Place all the ingredients in the blender and blend until the ice cubes are completely crushed.

CHOCOLATE-RASPBERRY SHAKE

> 1 serving chocolate-flavored soy protein powder
> 1 cup plain soy milk
> 1 cup frozen raspberries
> $1/8$ teaspoon orange extract
> 4 ice cubes

Place all the ingredients in the blender and blend until the ice cubes are completely crushed.

STRAWBERRY-KIWI SHAKE

 1 serving vanilla-flavored soy protein powder

 1 cup nonfat milk

 $^1/_2$ cup frozen whole strawberries

 1 very ripe kiwi, peeled

 $^1/_8$ teaspoon lemon extract

 4 ice cubes

Place all the ingredients in the blender and blend until the ice cubes are completely crushed.

CHAI TEA LATTE SMOOTHIE

 1 serving vanilla-flavored soy protein powder

 1 cup plain soy milk

 3 tablespoons unsweetened liquid iced tea concentrate

 $^1/_2$ medium banana

 Scant $^1/_8$ teaspoon cinnamon

 A few dashes each ginger, clove, black pepper

 4 to 5 ice cubes

Place all the ingredients in the blender and blend until the ice cubes are completely crushed.

BANANA-WALNUT SHAKE

 1 serving vanilla-flavored soy protein powder

 1 cup plain soy milk

 $^1/_2$ very ripe banana

 $^1/_8$ teaspoon black walnut flavoring

 Few drops vanilla extract

 Dash cinnamon

 4 ice cubes

Place all the ingredients in the blender and blend until the ice cubes are completely crushed.

PINEAPPLE-ORANGE-COCONUT SHAKE

    1 serving vanilla-flavored soy protein powder

    1 cup plain soy milk

    1 cup frozen pineapple chunks

    $\frac{1}{8}$ teaspoon coconut extract

    $\frac{1}{4}$ teaspoon orange extract

    4 ice cubes

Place all the ingredients in the blender and blend until the ice cubes are completely crushed.

VERY BERRY SHAKE

    1 serving vanilla-flavored soy protein powder

    $\frac{1}{3}$ cup nonfat dry milk powder

    1 cup low-calorie cranberry juice

    1 cup frozen mixed berries

    A few drops vanilla extract

    4 ice cubes

Place all the ingredients in the blender and blend until the ice cubes are completely crushed.

ORANGE-MANGO SHAKE

    1 serving vanilla-flavored soy protein powder

    1 cup nonfat milk or plain soy milk

    $\frac{1}{2}$ cup frozen mango chunks

    $\frac{1}{2}$ cup canned mandarin oranges, drained

    4 ice cubes

Place all the ingredients in the blender and blend until the ice cubes are completely crushed.

CHOCOLATE-STRAWBERRY SHAKE

> 1 serving scoop chocolate-flavored soy protein powder
>
> 1 cup nonfat milk or plain soy milk
>
> 1 cup frozen strawberries
>
> A few drops vanilla extract
>
> 4 ice cubes

Place all the ingredients in the blender and blend until the ice cubes are completely crushed.

ORANGE JULIUS SHAKE

> 1 serving vanilla-flavored soy protein powder
>
> 1 cup nonfat milk or plain soy milk
>
> 3 tablespoons frozen orange juice concentrate
>
> $1/4$ teaspoon vanilla extract
>
> 4 ice cubes

Place all the ingredients in the blender and blend until the ice cubes are completely crushed.

APPLE PIE SHAKE

> 1 serving vanilla-flavored soy protein powder
>
> 1 cup nonfat milk or plain soy milk
>
> 1 cup frozen apple slices
>
> A few dashes each cinnamon, nutmeg, cloves
>
> $1/4$ teaspoon vanilla extract
>
> 4 ice cubes

Place all the ingredients in the blender and blend until the ice cubes are completely crushed.

PEACH-ALMOND SHAKE

1 serving vanilla-flavored soy protein powder

1 cup nonfat milk or plain soy milk

1 cup frozen peach slices

A few dashes ground ginger

1/4 teaspoon almond extract

4 ice cubes

Place all the ingredients in the blender and blend thoroughly until the ice cubes are completely crushed.

CAFÉ MOCHA SHAKE

1 serving chocolate-flavored soy protein powder

1 cup nonfat milk or plain soy milk

2 teaspoons instant coffee crystals

1/2 medium banana

Dash cinnamon

4 ice cubes

Place all the ingredients in the blender and blend until the ice cubes are completely crushed.

BLUEBERRY-CRANBERRY SHAKE

1 scoop vanilla-flavored soy protein powder

1/3 cup nonfat dry milk

1 cup low calorie cranberry juice

1 cup frozen blueberries

A few drops orange extract

4 ice cubes

Place all the ingredients in the blender and blend until the ice cubes are completely crushed.

Activating Your Personal Plan

PINA COLADA SHAKE

1 scoop vanilla-flavored soy protein powder

1 cup plain soy milk

$^{1}/_{2}$ cup frozen pineapple chunks

$^{1}/_{4}$ small banana

$^{1}/_{4}$ teaspoon coconut extract

4 ice cubes

Place all the ingredients in the blender and blend until the ice cubes are completely crushed.

FRUIT- AND VEGETABLE-BASED SALAD DRESSINGS

These dressings are fat-free, but have a little more flavor and substance than plain vinegar or lemon—although with some meals a salad with just some fresh lemon juice, salt, and pepper hits the spot. Since the dressings contain fruits and vegetables, they provide a nutritional bonus, which most salad dressings do not. Don't be put off by the baby food ingredients—the pureed vegetables make the perfect flavoring base and thicken the dressings. If you like to experiment, try substituting different vinegars or lemon juice, and vary the herbs. You can double or triple these recipes; they will keep for at least a week in the refrigerator.

L.A. Shape Carrot Vinaigrette

MAKES ABOUT THREE 2-TABLESPOON SERVINGS

One 4-ounce jar baby-food carrots

3 tablespoons seasoned rice vinegar

1 tablespoon dried parsley flakes

$^{1}/_{2}$ teaspoon Worcestershire sauce

$^{1}/_{4}$ teaspoon dried basil

$^{1}/_{4}$ teaspoon dried oregano

$^1/_8$ teaspoon garlic powder

$^1/_4$ teaspoon salt

$^1/_4$ teaspoon pepper

Pour the baby-food carrots into a jar with a lid. Measure the rice vinegar into the empty baby-food jar, cover, shake to loosen the carrots, and pour the vinegar mixture into the other jar. Add the rest of the ingredients, shake well, and refrigerate.

Nutritional Analysis per Serving

Calories: 13; Protein: 0 grams; Fat: 0 grams; Carbohydrate: 3 grams

L.A. Shape "Green Goddess" Dressing

MAKES THREE 2-TABLESPOON SERVINGS

One 4-ounce jar baby-food green beans

3 tablespoons tarragon vinegar

1 teaspoon honey

$^1/_2$ teaspoon dried dill

$^1/_2$ teaspoon Dijon-style mustard

1 tablespoon dried parsley flakes

1 teaspoon dried chives

$^1/_4$ teaspoon pepper

$^1/_4$ teaspoon salt

Pour the baby-food green beans into a jar with a lid. Measure the vinegar into the empty baby-food jar, cover, shake to loosen the green beans, and pour the vinegar mixture into the other jar. Add the rest of the ingredients, shake well, and refrigerate.

Nutritional Analysis per Serving

Calories: 17; Protein: 0.5 gram; Fat: 0 gram; Carbohydrate: 4 grams

Activating Your Personal Plan

L.A. Shape Orange-Ginger Dressing

MAKES THREE 2-TABLESPOON SERVINGS

$^1/_4$ cup seasoned rice vinegar

1 tablespoon light soy sauce

2 teaspoons honey

$^1/_4$ teaspoon ground ginger

$^1/_8$ teaspoon white pepper

$^1/_4$ teaspoon wasabi (horseradish) powder

1 tablespoon sesame seeds

1 tablespoon dried chives

$^1/_4$ cup canned mandarin orange segments, drained

Place all the ingredients in the blender and blend thoroughly until smooth. Keep refrigerated for up to a week.

Nutritional Analysis per Serving

Calories: 43; Protein: 1 gram; Fat: 1.5 grams; Carbohydrate: 7 grams

Indian Chicken Curry with Cucumber Yogurt Salad

This spicy dish reheats well if you have any leftovers. Although it contains a fair number of ingredients, it comes together quickly. This is a basic recipe; feel free to experiment by adding other vegetables to the curry. The cool, refreshing side dish of cucumbers in yogurt provides terrific contrast to the spicy curry.

MAKES 4 SERVINGS

4 boneless, skinless chicken breast halves, cut into 1-inch cubes

Salt and pepper

Small amount of flour for dredging

Olive oil pan spray

2 teaspoons olive oil

1 medium onion, sliced

2 garlic cloves, chopped

One 14½-ounce can whole tomatoes

½ teaspoon hot red pepper flakes, or to taste

½ teaspoon ground coriander

1 teaspoon ground ginger

2 teaspoons curry powder

½ cup chopped fresh cilantro leaves

1 tablespoon fresh lemon juice

1. Sprinkle the chicken with salt and pepper, dredge lightly in flour, and set aside. Spray the inside of a medium stockpot with olive oil spray and place over medium-high heat. Add the olive oil.

2. Add the chicken pieces to the hot oil and sauté just until they start to brown, about 3 minutes. Add the onion and garlic, and sauté until the onions begin to soften, about 5 minutes. Add the tomatoes with their juice, red pepper flakes, coriander, ginger, and curry powder. Stir, cover, turn the heat to low, and simmer until the chicken is cooked through, about 15 minutes.

3. Before serving, adjust the seasonings and stir in the cilantro and lemon juice.

Nutritional Analysis per Serving
Calories: 220; Protein: 29 grams; Fat: 6 grams; Carbohydrate: 12 grams

CUCUMBER YOGURT SALAD

MAKES 4 SERVINGS

> 1½ cups plain nonfat yogurt
>
> 1 medium cucumber, peeled, seeded, and grated
>
> ½ teaspoon salt
>
> ½ teaspoon ground cumin
>
> ½ teaspoon sugar
>
> 2 tablespoons chopped fresh mint leaves *or* 2 teaspoons dried mint leaves

Combine all the ingredients in a medium bowl. Chill before serving.

Nutritional Analysis per Serving

Calories: 40; Protein: 4 grams; Fat: 0 gram; Carbohydrate: 6 grams

Asian Lettuce Cups

While many Asian restaurants serve lettuce cups as an appetizer, they make a delicious lunch or light dinner. Seasoned ground chicken breast, turkey breast, or soy "ground round" is spooned into crunchy lettuce leaves spread with a slightly sweet Hoisin sauce, found in most supermarkets with Asian cooking ingredients. This recipe is very flexible in that you can add any vegetables that you like. Just be sure to chop the vegetables into very small dice so they will cook quickly.

MAKES 3 SERVINGS

Sauce mixture

> 2 tablespoons oyster-flavored sauce*
>
> 2 tablespoons light soy sauce
>
> 1 tablespoon brown sugar
>
> ¼ teaspoon ground white pepper
>
> ¼ teaspoon ground ginger
>
> 2 teaspoons rice wine or dry sherry
>
> ¼ teaspoon garlic powder

Filling

> Olive oil pan spray
>
> 1 pound ground chicken breast or turkey breast, broken up
>
> 1 medium carrot, grated
>
> 1/3 cup canned water chestnuts, minced
>
> 2 green onions, chopped
>
> 1 small head Boston, Bibb, or romaine lettuce, outer leaves removed and inner leaves separated into about 9 "cups"
>
> Hoisin sauce*

1. Combine the sauce mixture ingredients in a small bowl and set aside.

2. Spray a large skillet with spray and place over high heat. Add the chicken or turkey and sauté, breaking up the meat with a wooden spoon, until it is no longer pink, 4 to 5 minutes. If there is liquid in the skillet, drain it off. Set the meat aside in a bowl.

3. Wipe the pan with a paper towel, spray it again with olive oil spray, and return to high heat. Add the carrot, water chestnuts, and green onions, and stir-fry until the vegetables are just beginning to soften, about 1 minute. Return the meat to the pan, mix well, and pour in the sauce mixture. Stir until the meat is evenly coated.

4. To serve, spoon about a teaspoon of Hoisin sauce on each lettuce leaf, top with the meat mixture, roll up the lettuce, and enjoy.

*Available in most supermarkets in the Asian foods section.

Nutritional Analysis per Serving
Calories: 225; Protein: 37 grams; Fat: 3 grams; Carbohydrate: 12 grams

Quick Chicken Soup

Most chicken soups are light on the chicken. This quick soup serves as a whole meal because it contains plenty of chicken to supply healthy, low-fat protein. Vegetables freshen the broth and give it a true homemade flavor in a fraction of the time a homemade soup would require. Feel free to add other vegetables that appeal to you. The grated zucchini substitutes for the higher-calorie noodles that typically fill up the soup bowl.

MAKES 4 GENEROUS SERVINGS

> Three 14½-ounce cans reduced-sodium chicken broth
>
> 1 small onion, halved and thinly sliced
>
> 1 carrot, cut into ¼-inch dice
>
> 1 celery stalk, cut into ¼-inch dice
>
> 1 teaspoon instant chicken bouillon granules
>
> Dash of nutmeg
>
> Pepper to taste
>
> Two 10-ounce cans chicken breast meat, liquid drained, meat flaked with a fork
>
> 2 medium zucchini, unpeeled and grated
>
> 2 tablespoons chopped fresh or 1 tablespoon dried parsley flakes

1. In a medium stockpot, combine the chicken broth, onion, carrot, celery, bouillon granules, nutmeg, and pepper. Bring to a boil over high heat, reduce to low, cover, and simmer until vegetables are just tender, 5 to 6 minutes. Raise the heat to medium, add the chicken, and heat through, about 2 minutes.

2. Turn off the heat and add the zucchini and parsley. Cover and let stand for a few minutes, until the zucchini is heated through. Adjust the seasonings and serve.

Nutritional Analysis per Serving

Calories: 200; Protein: 38 grams; Fat: 2 grams; Carbohydrate: 6 grams

Juicy Roast Turkey Breast

Turkey breast roasted in the oven is often dry. Try this stovetop method and you may never roast turkey breast in the oven again. The meat is flavorful and moist—great as a hot entrée and terrific the next day diced into a salad for a quick meal. You will need a heavy casserole or Dutch oven with a tight-fitting lid.

MAKES 6 GENEROUS SERVINGS

> Olive oil pan spray
> 1 fresh breast half of turkey (2 to 2½ pounds), rinsed and patted dry
> 1 teaspoon olive oil
> 2 tablespoons white wine or water
> ¼ cup reduced sodium chicken or vegetable stock
> 1 medium onion, cut in half and sliced
> ¼ teaspoon salt
> Ground black pepper to taste
> ½ teaspoon dried thyme or 2 teaspoons fresh thyme leaves

1. Make sure your heavy casserole or Dutch oven is large enough to hold the turkey breast. Spray the pan with olive oil spray. Spray the turkey breast lightly with olive oil spray.

2. Place the casserole over medium-high heat and add the olive oil. When the oil is hot, place the turkey breast in the casserole, skin side down, and let it brown, about 5 minutes. Remove the turkey to a plate and set aside.

3. Lower the heat to medium-low and add the white wine or water and stock to deglaze the pan. Stir with a wooden spoon to loosen any browned bits. Add the onion, salt, and pepper, and stir until the onions begin to soften, about 3 minutes.

4. Place the turkey, skin side down, on top of the onion. Cover tightly and cook about 45 minutes, turning the turkey skin side up halfway through cooking. There should be about ¼ cup of liquid in the bottom of the casserole; add water a few tablespoons at a time as needed.

5. The turkey is done when the internal temperature reaches 180°F. Slice and serve with the pan juices drizzled on top.

Nutritional Analysis per Serving
Calories: 230; Protein: 43 grams; Fat: 4 grams; Carbohydrate: 2 grams

Roasted Eggplant Salad

If you are fond of roasted vegetables, you will like this salad. Roasting the eggplant gives it a delicious smoky flavor, and while this dish may be unusual to American palates, it is served all over the Mediterranean in various forms as a side dish to fish and poultry. You can serve this as a first course salad, as a side dish to your entrée, or you can add roasted chicken or diced grilled tofu to the salad for a one-dish meal.

MAKES ABOUT 5 SERVINGS

Olive oil pan spray
2 eggplants
1 teaspoon salt
4 tablespoons fresh lemon juice
2 teaspoons olive oil
2 medium tomatoes, diced
1 garlic clove, minced
1 tablespoon minced parsley
Ground black pepper to taste

1. Preheat the broiler. Cover a baking sheet with aluminum foil and spray lightly with pan spray.

2. Cut the stem end off the eggplants, then cut them in half lengthwise and place, cut side down, on the prepared cookie sheet. Place under the broiler, about 3 inches away from the heat, and broil until the skins are blackened and the flesh is very soft when you pierce the eggplants with a fork. This should take about 20 minutes.

3. Remove the eggplants from the oven and allow to cool until you can handle them. Scrape the eggplant flesh into a medium mixing bowl and discard the skins. The flesh should be very soft and should come away from the skin easily. With a large fork, whip and mash the eggplant to smooth it somewhat. Add the remaining ingredients and mix well, adjusting seasonings to your taste.

4. You can serve this salad at room temperature, or refrigerate and eat cold.

Nutritional Analysis per Serving
Calories: 40; Protein: 1 gram; Fat: 2 grams; Carbohydrate: 6 grams

Baja Seafood Cocktail

This seafood cocktail makes a great main dish on a warm summer evening. The spicy fish and vegetable mix is light yet filling. The avocado should be somewhat firm for this dish; if it's too ripe it may fall apart and spoil the appearance of the cocktail. Make this in midsummer when fresh tomatoes are at their peak, and serve with a tossed salad sweetened with mandarin oranges or mango chunks.

MAKES 4 SERVINGS

1 pound frozen cooked shrimp

1/2 pound imitation crab flakes

3 medium tomatoes, cut into small dice

1 cucumber, peeled, seeds removed and cut into small dice

2 garlic cloves, minced

1/4 cup chopped cilantro leaves

1/3 cup prepared ketchup

1/3 cup water

1/2 teaspoon salt

1 teaspoon ground cumin

1/2 teaspoon liquid hot pepper sauce, or to taste

Juice of 2 fresh limes

1 avocado, diced

1. Place the frozen shrimp in a strainer and run under cool water for a few minutes to separate them and allow them to begin to thaw. Put the imitation crab in the same strainer and run under cool water briefly, separating the pieces into shreds. Set aside.

2. In a large serving bowl, stir together the tomatoes, cucumber, garlic, cilantro, ketchup, water, salt, cumin, liquid hot pepper sauce, and lime juice. Once well mixed, gently stir in the seafood and finally the diced avocado. The shrimp will continue to thaw in the mixture and make the cocktail very cold.

3. Once the shrimp is defrosted, the cocktail is ready to serve. If you plan to serve later, refrigerate until serving.

Nutritional Analysis per Serving
Calories: 292; Protein: 33 grams; Fat: 10 grams; Carbohydrate: 20 grams

Jamaican Spiced Chicken

A plain baked or broiled chicken breast can get boring, but the great thing about it is that it takes on the flavors of a marinade so well. This recipe is similar to "jerked" chicken, which is a traditional Jamaican method of preserving and roasting meats with dry spice rubs and spicy marinades. It's convenient to marinate the chicken in the refrigerator during the day and come home to a quick meal. Try this dish with a fruit salsa on the side and a tossed salad. This flavorful chicken is great cold the next day, too.

MAKES 4 SERVINGS

> 3 tablespoons ground allspice
> 1 teaspoon ground cinnamon
> ½ teaspoon ground nutmeg
> 1 tablespoon ground coriander
> 2 garlic cloves, minced

2 tablespoons frozen orange juice concentrate

2 teaspoons olive oil

$\frac{1}{2}$ teaspoon salt

$\frac{1}{2}$ teaspoon black pepper

$\frac{1}{4}$ teaspoon hot red pepper flakes

4 large boneless chicken breast halves, skin removed

1. In a bowl large enough to hold the chicken breasts, combine the allspice, cinnamon, nutmeg, coriander, garlic, orange juice concentrate, olive oil, salt, pepper, and chile flakes. If the mixture seems too dry to spread, add a few teaspoons of water. Blend well. Add the chicken breasts and stir gently with a rubber spatula to coat. Transfer the chicken and marinade to a plastic storage bag, seal tightly, and place in the refrigerator several hours or overnight.

2. You will need a lidded skillet large enough to hold the chicken pieces. Spray the skillet with olive oil spray and heat it over medium-high heat. When hot, add the chicken and brown on one side, about 3 minutes. Turn the chicken pieces over, cover the skillet, turn the heat to low, and cook the chicken until it's done, about 10 minutes. The chicken pieces can also be grilled on the barbecue until done, about 10 minutes.

Nutritional Analysis per Serving
Calories: 200; Protein: 33 grams; Fat: 5 grams; Carbohydrate: 4 grams

Gazpacho

This is a great soup to make during the summer, when fresh tomatoes are at their peak from the garden or the farmers' market. You can make this with canned tomatoes, too—the soup won't be quite as thick, but it's still delicious. This recipe makes a large amount, and it's great to have in the refrigerator for a quick, low-calorie snack.

MAKES 8 GENEROUS SERVINGS

5 whole tomatoes, cored and sliced

3 garlic cloves

2 teaspoons salt

2 teaspoons ground cumin

$^1/_4$ teaspoon Tabasco sauce

1 teaspoon pepper

1 tablespoon olive oil

1 teaspoon Worcestershire sauce

$^1/_3$ cup tarragon vinegar

One 46-ounce can tomato juice

$^1/_2$ cup chopped green onion

$^1/_2$ cup chopped green bell pepper

$^1/_2$ cup chopped celery

$^1/_2$ cup chopped cucumber

1. Place the first 9 ingredients in the blender and blend until smooth. Pour the mixture into a large bowl and stir in the rest of the ingredients.

2. Chill well and serve very cold.

Nutritional Analysis per Serving

Calories: 67; Protein: 2 grams; Fat: 2 grams; Carbohydrate: 12 grams

Thai-Style Scallops with Basil

This recipe isn't difficult, but it has some unusual flavors. Thai fish sauce is quite widely available in most supermarkets that carry Asian ingredients. If you're not a fan of scallops, substitute shrimp or chicken breasts.

MAKES 2 SERVINGS

1 pound scallops, fresh or frozen, defrosted

2 tablespoons Thai fish sauce (nam pla)*

1 tablespoon light soy sauce

1 tablespoon sugar

Olive oil spray

2 teaspoons olive oil

1 tablespoon minced garlic

$\frac{1}{2}$ teaspoon hot red pepper flakes

1 medium red bell pepper, cut into thin strips

1 medium carrot, cut into thin matchsticks

1 cup fresh basil leaves

1. In a medium bowl, combine the scallops, fish sauce, soy sauce, water, and sugar. Set aside.

2. Spray a large nonstick frying pan with olive oil spray, add the olive oil, and heat over medium-high heat. Add the garlic and cook, stirring, for 1 minute. Stir in the red pepper flakes, red bell pepper, and carrot, and cook, stirring, for 1 minute.

3. With a slotted spoon, remove the scallops from the marinade and add them to the hot pan. Cook and stir until the scallops are almost done, about 3 minutes. Add the marinade and cook 1 minute, stirring to coat the scallops and vegetables.

4. Remove from the heat and stir in the fresh basil.

*Usually available in the Asian section of most supermarkets.

Nutritional Analysis per Serving
Calories: 300; Protein: 40 grams; Fat: 6.5 grams; Carbohydrate: 19 grams

Sherry-Braised Chicken and Mushrooms

This is a quick and healthy recipe similar to chicken in wine sauce, but the recipe does not produce a large amount of sauce. Instead, the chicken tenders are browned and then glazed with just enough sherry to coat them attractively and keep them moist.

MAKES 3 SERVINGS

Flour for dredging

1 pound chicken breast tenders

Salt and pepper

Olive oil spray

½ pound fresh mushrooms, thinly sliced

1 small onion, halved and thinly sliced

1 celery stalk, thinly sliced on the diagonal

2 tablespoons low-sodium chicken broth

3 tablespoons dry sherry

½ teaspoon dried tarragon

1. Spread a small amount of flour on a flat work surface. Dip the chicken tenders in flour on both sides and set them aside on a plate. Sprinkle with salt and pepper.

2. Spray a large skillet with olive oil spray and heat it over medium-high heat. Add the chicken in a single layer and brown on one side, about 3 minutes. Turn the pieces over, spraying the pan with additional spray if necessary to prevent sticking, and brown the other side, about 3 minutes. Set the chicken aside on a plate.

3. Add the mushrooms, onion, celery, and broth, and cook, scraping up any browned bits on the bottom of the skillet, until the vegetables are just tender, about 3 minutes. Add the sherry and tarragon, and raise the heat to high. Cook, stirring constantly, until the sauce is reduced and thick enough to coat the chicken pieces, about 2 minutes.

4. Return the chicken to the pan and stir gently to coat with the glaze.

Nutritional Analysis per Serving
Calories: 230; Protein: 38 grams; Fat: 2.5 grams; Carbohydrate: 13 grams

Oven-"Fried" Fish

There are lots of recipes for oven-fried fish. And no wonder—it's such a great technique for keeping fish moist on the inside and crispy on the outside, with almost no added fat. This recipe is quick and takes advantage of a packaged dry sauce mix. While the lemon sauce mix is a natural with fish, feel free to experiment. Chicken taco seasoning mix makes a spicier, but equally delicious, fish.

MAKES 2 SERVINGS

> 1 pound cod or snapper fillets, rinsed under cool water and patted dry
> ¼ cup nonfat milk
> 2 egg whites
> ½ cup plain dried bread crumbs
> 2 tablespoons lemon chicken sauce mix powder
> Lemon slices for garnish

1. Preheat the oven to 475°F. Spray a baking dish large enough to hold the fillets in a single layer with olive oil spray.

2. In a wide, shallow bowl, mix the milk and egg whites with a fork until well blended. On a plate, combine the bread crumbs and sauce mix with your fingers until well blended. Dip the fillets first in the egg white mixture and then in the bread crumb mixture, coating well on both sides.

3. Place the fish in the baking dish and spray the top of the fish lightly with olive oil spray. Bake until fish flakes easily with a fork, about 20 minutes. Serve garnished with fresh lemon.

Nutritional Analysis per Serving
Calories: 388; Protein: 60 grams; Fat: 5 grams; Carbohydrate: 21 grams

Chicken and Turkey Meat Loaf

This meat loaf is juicy and delicious. A large loaf would generally take at least an hour and a half to cook in a conventional oven, but this one is precooked in the microwave, which cuts the total cooking time in half. It will be paler than regular meat loaf, but the flavor is terrific—and it has much less fat than a traditional loaf. It also tastes great cold—just slice it on top of a salad.

MAKES 8 SERVINGS

Activating Your Personal Plan

Olive oil spray

2 egg whites

$\frac{1}{4}$ cup nonfat milk

$\frac{1}{2}$ cup seasoned bread crumbs

1 tablespoon bottled steak sauce (such as A.1.)

2 tablespoons ketchup

$\frac{1}{2}$ medium onion, grated

1 carrot, grated

$1\frac{1}{2}$ teaspoons salt

$\frac{1}{2}$ teaspoon ground black pepper

$\frac{1}{2}$ teaspoon dried thyme

$\frac{1}{2}$ teaspoon garlic powder

2 teaspoons dried parsley flakes

1 pound each ground chicken and turkey breast *or* 2 pounds ground turkey breast

1. Preheat the oven to 325°F. Spray an 8-inch square oven-safe dish with olive oil spray.

2. In a bowl large enough to hold the meat, beat the eggs whites and milk. Add the bread crumbs, steak sauce, and ketchup, and mix well with a fork. Let stand for 5 minutes, or until the bread crumbs have absorbed the liquid. Stir in the onion, carrot, salt, pepper, thyme, garlic powder, and parsley. Add the ground meat and mix thoroughly with clean hands.

3. Turn the mixture into the prepared baking dish and shape it into a loaf. Spray the top with olive oil spray. Microwave on high for 25 minutes, then transfer to the oven and bake for 25 minutes.

4. Let the meat loaf rest out of the oven for 10 minutes so that it will slice more easily.

Nutritional Analysis per Serving

Calories: 175; Protein: 28 grams; Fat: 2 grams; Carbohydrate: 9 grams

Creamy Butternut Squash Soup

Butternut squash soup is a beautiful orange color because it is naturally rich in beta-carotene. You can usually find frozen diced squash in the supermarket, which makes this a very quick soup to put together. The addition of the tofu makes the soup creamy with very little fat, and adds a protein boost.

MAKES 6 SERVINGS

> 4 cups canned vegetable broth
> 2 large onions, diced
> 2 pounds peeled and diced butternut squash
> 1 pound soft tofu, drained and diced
> 1 teaspoon ground ginger
> 1 tablespoon lemon juice
> $\frac{1}{2}$ teaspoon dried thyme
> 1 teaspoon salt
> Freshly ground black pepper to taste
> Fresh thyme or thin strips of lemon peel for garnish, if desired

1. In a large pot over medium heat, heat $\frac{1}{4}$ cup of the vegetable broth. Add the onions and cook until tender, about 3 minutes. Add the squash and the remaining vegetable broth. Bring to a boil over medium-high heat, reduce the heat to low, and simmer, uncovered, until the squash is very tender, about 20 minutes. Add the tofu and ginger, lemon juice, thyme, salt, and pepper, and simmer until the tofu is heated through, about 2 minutes.

2. In a blender or food processor, purée the soup in batches. Return to the pan and reheat until the soup is very hot but not boiling.

3. Ladle the soup into bowls and garnish with the fresh thyme or lemon peel, if desired.

Nutritional Analysis per Serving
Calories: 155; Protein: 10 grams; Fat: 3 grams; Carbohydrate: 25 grams

Quick California Rolls

California rolls are popular in sushi bars because crab and avocado go so wonderfully together. The problem is that they are loaded with starchy white rice, and sometimes even have mayonnaise added to the crabmeat mixture. This version uses long, flat strips of cucumber to enclose the crab and avocado filling. They look pretty served on their sides so that you can see the spiral filling.

MAKES 2 SERVINGS

> 2 large cucumbers
> ½ medium avocado, pitted and peeled
> ½ teaspoon wasabi (horseradish) powder
> 1 teaspoon soy sauce
> ½ teaspoon ground ginger
> 1 teaspoon lemon juice
> 12 ounces imitation crabmeat, rinsed under running water and flaked with your fingers
> 1 carrot, grated
> Pickled ginger and wasabi paste as an accompaniment, if desired

1. Peel the cucumbers and slice them lengthwise as thinly as possible, like lasagna noodles. Set the slices aside on a plate.

2. Place the avocado in a medium bowl and mash it with a fork. Add the wasabi powder, soy sauce, ground ginger, and lemon juice and mix well. Add the crabmeat and mix well.

3. To assemble, spread the crab/avocado mixture on the cucumber strips, top with some grated carrot, and roll it up. Secure the roll with a toothpick. Stand the rolls on their sides on the serving plate so that the filling shows.

Nutritional Analysis per Serving
Calories: 225; Protein: 22 grams; Fat: 10 grams; Carbohydrate: 26 grams

Healthy Cabbage Slaw

Deli-style coleslaw is heavy on the mayonnaise, which is too bad because it really masks the flavor of the cabbage. This version features cabbage and carrots and a spicy dressing made with Anaheim chile. The dressing is great on regular salad greens, too.

MAKES 12 SERVINGS

> 1 small head green cabbage
> 2 large carrots, grated
> 1/4 cup minced parsley

Dressing

> 1 whole canned mild green Anaheim chile
> 1/2 cup tarragon or rice wine vinegar
> 1 tablespoon lime juice
> 2 tablespoons olive oil
> 1 tablespoon Dijon-style mustard
> 1/2 teaspoon garlic powder
> 2 teaspoons sugar
> 1 1/4 teaspoons salt
> 1/2 teaspoon ground cumin
> 1/4 teaspoon Tabasco sauce
> Freshly ground black pepper to taste

1. Core the cabbage and discard the tough outer leaves. Cut the cabbage in half and shred it into very fine strips. Place it in a colander and rinse under very hot water, squeezing gently until it softens slightly, about 2 minutes. Rinse with cold water. Working in large handfuls, place the cabbage in a kitchen towel and pat it dry. As you finish with each handful, place the cabbage in a large bowl. Add the carrots and parsley, and toss.

2. Put all the dressing ingredients in the blender and blend until smooth. Add to cabbage mixture and toss thoroughly.

3. Chill well to allow the flavors to blend before serving.

Nutritional Analysis per Serving
Calories: 53; Protein: 1 gram; Fat: 2 grams; Carbohydrate: 8 grams

Quick Soy Chili

If you haven't experimented much with soy meat substitutes, this is a great place to start. Soy ground meat "crumbles" work particularly well to replace ground meats in highly seasoned dishes like this one. The chopped vegetables replace the higher-calorie beans and add texture and nutrition. If you want to make this dish even easier, you can replace all the seasonings with a package of taco seasoning mix. The chili is good on its own with a salad, Healthy Cabbage Slaw (page 127), or vegetables on the side; or if you're a fan of taco salad, you can put a scoop on top of mixed greens and enjoy it as a one-dish meal.

MAKES 6 SERVINGS

> Olive oil spray
> 1 medium onion, chopped
> 1 carrot, diced
> 2 celery stalks, chopped
> One 4-ounce can diced mild green chiles
> Two 14½-ounce cans stewed tomatoes (1 can puréed in the blender)
> 2 packages soy ground meat substitute, about 12 ounces each
> 1 teaspoon ground cumin
> 1 teaspoon dried oregano leaves
> 2 tablespoons ground chili powder
> 1 teaspoon salt
> ¼ teaspoon liquid hot pepper sauce
> Fresh cilantro leaves for garnish, optional

1. Spray a medium stockpot with olive oil spray and place it over medium-high heat. Add the onion, carrot, and celery, and sauté until the vegetables begin to soften, about 5 minutes. Add the 2 cans of tomatoes (puréed and not puréed), soy meat substitute, and seasonings. Stir well and bring to a boil.

2. Cover, lower the heat to medium-low, and simmer until the flavors are blended, 15 to 20 minutes.

3. Garnish with fresh cilantro, if desired.

Nutritional Analysis Per Serving:

Calories: 180; Protein: 22 grams; Fat: 2 grams; Carbohydrate: 22 grams

Reinforce Your Habits

The Art of Relapse Prevention

The hardest thing in life is to change your established habits, even when you know those habits are causing you problems. Human behavior is not like a light switch that you can turn on and off at will. Any habit goes away slowly, and you can count on making mistakes.

Lapse-Relapse-Collapse

A single mistake is a lapse, and we are all entitled to lapses as we try to learn a new habit. A string of lapses or the regular and repeated occurrences of lapses is called a relapse. If unchecked, relapses evolve into collapse, or giving up entirely on your mission to change. Research has shown that the best place to stop the chain of lapse-relapse-collapse is to try to prevent relapses. In this chapter you will learn about relapse prevention by understanding the behaviors that have you stuck in a rut right now.

We are all creatures of habit. It is in our genes. Childhood is prolonged in humans, in comparison to all other animals, in order to give us the chance to master all the many different things we need to know as adults. This learning is accomplished through a process of repetition. Children take pleasure in repetition; they love games they can play over and over again and songs with repetitive verses. When you repeat an old habit, your body reacts positively. Changing habits is hard and takes effort.

Simple examples from everyday life are easy to find. In a lecture hall, people usually take the same seat after a break—even when those seats are not assigned in any way, and even when they're attending a single lecture, not part of a class. In the same way, some people open a can of beer as soon as they get home or unconsciously eat pretzels or chips when they are stressed.

People in the food industry know this, and that is why they will do almost anything to get you to form the habit of buying their products. Once such habits are formed, they know that you won't easily stop getting them. That is what brand loyalty is all about. There are great examples of battles in which companies fight for the loyalty of customers consuming very similar products. A coupon that promises a "buy one, get one free" offer is just one of many ways to get you to try a new product (and, by extension, to reject a competitor's product). Once you have bought a food product and tasted it, they've almost got you. The rest of the work is done by your programmed reaction to triggers in your environment that are part of the positioning of the advertised product. So the next thing you know, you are consuming the product not only for its taste, but to be part of a cool generation or to mimic your favorite athlete (whether or not the athlete actually touches the stuff in real life!). The color and design of the wrapper also plays into that image. A lot of work goes into getting you hooked.

Antecedents, Behaviors, Consequences

In order to break a habit, you must become aware of what triggers your behaviors. Your food habits are much more than simply an attraction to tastes that you find pleasant. They are triggered by certain emotions or situations in your life.

A repeated behavior or habit can be broken down into "ABC's": an-

tecedents, behaviors, and consequences. An antecedent is an event that occurs before a behavior and is linked to that behavior. For example, in classi-
cal experiments, a rat learns to associate a a green light (antecedent) with a
behavior (pulling a lever) and gets food (the consequence). However, if he
sees a red light (antecedent) and pulls the lever (behavior), he will get an
electrical shock (a different and unpleasant consequence). After a short period of training, the rat will consistently pull the green lever for food. Like
the rat, you may have learned that when you are upset (antecedent) you feel
the need to eat some chocolate ice cream (behavior) to make yourself feel
better (consequence). While this is a short-term pleasant consequence, the
long-term outcome is weight gain which, like the electrical shock to the rat,
is unpleasant. So in the case of your eating habits, it is important to disso-
ciate stress from eating and associate it with a healthy habit, such as taking
a walk or a meditation/relaxation break. Here the consequence will be reduction of your stress without the weight gain that comes from trying to
reduce your stress by eating. What are your ABC's?

When you look closely at your eating habits, you will find that you
sometimes consume food without tasting or appreciating it. These un-
scheduled eating events often undercut your efforts at losing weight. If you
drink your protein shakes diligently, you won't be hungry, but you'll still be
subject to cravings for Trigger Foods whenever they are put in front of you.
There are several ways to change this pattern.

First of all, you can become aware of the circumstances surrounding
your uncontrolled eating behaviors. By avoiding those times and places,
you can prevent the overeating and the sense that you've lost control. These
circumstances set you up for the behavior you are trying to avoid, so instead of feeling like a victim, take charge and change what this book calls
antecedents. These antecedents fall into one of two categories: things you

can change and things you can't change. But even if you can't change some of the antecedents that are driving you to overeat, you can change your reaction to them. Here are four steps, each starting with the letter S, that I learned from Dr. John Foreyt, who directs the nutrition program at Baylor University in Texas.

STRESS REDUCTION

You can attack your eating-related stress indirectly by reducing your overall stress level. Reading a novel, taking time to exercise, sleeping better, and making yourself a priority are all ways to decrease your overall stress level. Taking a walk instead of raiding the refrigerator may do more to reduce stress than eating a whole box of cookies. In fact, studies show that 92 percent of those who maintain their weight loss exercise regularly, while only 34 percent of those who regain lost weight exercise regularly. (See Step 6 for some advice on exercise.)

STIMULUS CONTROL

Here's an example: You awake to find a cold floor by your bed in the morning. To avoid this problem in the future, you place some bedroom slippers by your bed before retiring. The next morning you wake up and there are the slippers waiting for you. As a result, the cold floor doesn't bother you anymore. In dietary terms, this may mean stocking your refrigerator with healthy foods and getting rid of unhealthy foods, or it may mean planning what you will eat at an event. I often advise my patients to drink a high-protein shake before they go to a wedding, for example, and then eat selectively from the salad and vegetables, while only tasting the rubber chicken stuffed with cheese or the steak wrapped in bacon.

SELF-MONITORING

Use a journal or calendar every day to keep track of your efforts to control your eating. After each positive week, put a reward aside for yourself in the future.

SOCIAL SUPPORT

Stay away from people who criticize you for being overweight, and seek out those who will say positive things as you lose weight. Many people will want you to regain your weight for various reasons—and they may not even admit it to themselves. Some people may simply be envious; seeing you lose weight makes them uncomfortable about their own weight. A spouse may be threatened by your weight loss because he or she fears that you will now attract attention from the opposite sex. If you have a close friend who has a very positive attitude, consider working together on your weight-loss efforts. It is more fun to walk with a partner, and you can work through this book with a partner! You can lean on each other for support; communities on the Internet, such as the one offered at www.LAShape Diet.com, are another way to get social support.

FOUR STEPS TO PREVENT ANTECEDENTS FROM LEADING TO BEHAVIORS

Antecedents ⟶ Behaviors

Stress Reduction

Stimulus Control

Self-monitoring

Social Support

Now, let's deal with the behavior itself. You can change the nature of the behavior by eating better foods or smaller portions. So you may give yourself permission to eat off of your diet—perhaps for the one meal you eat every Sunday night at your mother's house. However, you can choose wisely and eat smaller portions while there. Finally, even if you cannot prevent an episode of overeating, you can change the consequences of that behavior by compensating for it with healthy behaviors. Let's say you have had a wonderful weekend and indulged in lots of delicious, heavy meals. Now you are back at work. Why not use two meal replacements a day for four days and see if you can make up for the extra calories you had over the weekend? Then go back to your one meal replacement a day. There is no guilt or anger when you exercise the option to correct your ABC's on your own. By understanding how you can use the ABC's, you'll have a new power over your body. But no one is perfect, so the consequences you don't want will happen. However, bad consequences in terms of weight gain never result from messing up just once or twice. It is really collections of ABC's forming a behavior pattern that will undo your efforts. In the next section, you will learn how to deal with the behaviors that don't work out the way you planned.

Coping Strategies

Even if you can't prevent a lapse, you can change your way of reacting to the lapse. First, you have to be able to ask yourself why the lapse occurred *without* getting down on yourself. Almost everyone will have lapses at one time or another. Try to observe your situation and identify the problem. Getting mad at yourself will only make things worse, so stay calm and collected. Second, renew your commitment in self-talk or writing. Self-talk is talking to yourself in a way that is meant to change your behavior patterns. Remind yourself why losing weight is so important to you. Revisit your goals. Tell yourself it would be ridiculous to abandon all your hard work now over just one little lapse. Get right back on your program. Don't use the lapse as an excuse to quit. Finally, get social support by discussing your problems with a professional, a friend, a support group, or an Internet pal. Coping with the inevitable slips is as important as putting a process of relapse prevention into place.

Relapse Prevention

The theory of relapse prevention comes from addiction psychology research. It is well known that smokers who try to quit often do so repeatedly. Mark Twain is quoted as saying that he quit smoking ten times. Humans are imperfect, and you cannot abandon your resolve every time you make a mistake. There will be times when you simply go off your plan. To keep this from happening repeatedly, you need to write down your lapses and find out whether they fall into a particular pattern.

Do you always buy fast food on the way home from work? Is it because you are hungry and haven't planned a healthy meal that you can make at home? The answer is to have your kitchen set up for easy food preparation. Buy frozen meals or frozen chicken breasts or fish and defrost them in the refrigerator before you leave for work in the morning. Put the meat on the grill, or use an electric low-fat grill that drains off excess fat, and steam some frozen vegetables in a microwave. Add a packaged salad, and you are all set to have a quick and easy meal when you get home. If you need something to tide you over while you drive home, carry a protein bar with you.

Relapse prevention uses the tools discussed previously in the section on ABC's in an intense, directed way when your behaviors are at their greatest risk of going out of control. By recognizing your lapses and doing something about them, you are preventing relapses and ultimate collapse. Relapse prevention involves seeing a pattern in your behavior that needs to be changed and changing it before it goes out of control.

Get Set, Get Ready, Go, Relax, Start Over

I recently saw a cartoon in the *New Yorker* that showed a middle-aged woman sitting with her two friends at a restaurant. As she is lifting a forkful of chocolate cake to her mouth, she says, "I set a goal, I met it, I proved that I could meet it, and now the hell with it." Believe it or not, I think this is healthy behavior. Give yourself permission to let loose once in a while. For some people, one night off per week to treat themselves to a meal they want is all the reward they need to stay on course.

Changing behavior is not easy, so first set a goal and a date to start. Then get ready by buying what you need and putting it in place. Now, go to it. Use all your determination to meet your goal.

SETTING GOALS YOU CAN ACHIEVE

Weekly Weight Loss _____

Eating Behavior _____

Exercise _____

Fun and Leisure _____

Family _____

Job _____

Other _____

A common problem is setting unrealistic goals that no one can achieve. This will just discourage you. You should know about how much weight you can realistically lose each week, and that can be one goal. However, it shouldn't be your only goal. If you are having trouble getting rid of a certain Trigger Food habit, see if you can reduce the behavior by half one week and then eliminate it altogether the next week. Try slowing down your eating by putting your fork down between bites. You can take an additional 5 or 10 minutes to eat your meal, or take a break of 10 minutes between courses. Eat your salad first, and then take a break. Sit down and eat the main meal, and then take a break. Then eat your fruit for dessert.

Keep track of your progress on these smaller goals, and you will know that you are moving toward your ultimate goal of losing weight and keeping it off for a lifetime. Reward yourself for achieving this goal, but now it is time to start over. Set another goal and go for that one. You need to make step-by-step changes, but there is always more you can do and more you can learn. I believe the best defense is a good offense, and not just in football. If you concentrate on meeting your next goal, you won't have the time to worry about losing ground on the goal you have already achieved.

Self-Talk

Self-talk is such an important strategy that I want to review what it means again and how to use it in detail. When you are in the middle of trying to change a behavior, self-talk can help you follow through with your intentions. This self-talk is not talking out loud, but rather listening to a voice within.

If I am approaching a buffet table and see a lot of foods that I should not be eating, I can use self-talk to convince myself that I really don't want those foods. I think about how many hours on the treadmill one piece of chocolate cake represents. I look carefully at fatty foods to find disgusting aspects of the food, such as pools of oil or grease spots on the table. I use enough negative imaging to outweigh my desire for the food. I also focus on how great the right foods will taste—for example, how refreshing the cantaloupe or watermelon will be.

Sometimes you just have to say no using self-talk. I remember flying in business class on airlines when dessert was an ice cream sundae made any way you wanted it. I could hear the wagon loaded with hot fudge sundaes coming down the aisle. I started talking to myself, saying no, no, no for several minutes, reminding myself of the resolve to say no. As the cart passed, I was still saying no to myself in a loud inner voice. If you did nothing and waited for the stewardess to put the ice cream in front of your face, I daresay there would be at least a 50 percent chance you might say yes, just this one time. The key to self-talk is to plan beforehand what you want to say to yourself to get the desired results.

Write It Down

For many people, the most effective way to get their feelings under control is to see them in writing. Writing down how you feel can be such a valuable tool that it is worth going over in more detail here. If writing down lists and feelings is something you like to do, then keeping a daily journal is a great way to stay on course. Writing down everything you eat and the exercise you do can be a very effective way of keeping track of your behaviors. I like to review one week at a time and use Sunday nights to plan the next week. You can find your own best routine, but get a journal and start writing things down. What behaviors do you want to change each day? When did you lapse, and why? How might you react differently the next time under the same circumstances?

We all want kudos for our accomplishments, and you can give them to yourself in writing. Write down the behaviors that you want to applaud, and give yourself a star when you have completed them. At the end of the week add up the stars and give yourself a weekly reward score. Set a goal for accomplishing a number of star points in order to earn a nonfood reward. You can save money for this reward by not buying all the foods that you shouldn't be eating and by skipping fast food meals. You will find that meal replacements cost less than the foods they replace.

Recognizing and Changing Patterns of Behavior

By looking at your journal, you may be able to see patterns of behaviors. You may be munching in the afternoon at work or at night in front of the television. You may have been having a great week until your boss yelled at you. Look at your behavior patterns and analyze them in terms of timing, probable aggravating factors, and direct triggers to either healthy or unhealthy behaviors.

How Not to Rain on Your Own Parade

Have you ever wondered why you seem to act against your own interests? It may seem that you have everything under control when, for no clear reason, you sabotage yourself. There are many reasons for self-destructive behaviors, including fear of changing. I have had many female patients who sabotaged their weight-loss efforts because they did not welcome the attention that they got from men after losing weight. These women were using their fat as a shield against having to face their fear of a relationship with a man. In these cases, discussing relationship issues in individual or group therapy helped these women conquer their fear of relationships, and their weight loss followed. Mild depression can also be a reason for sabotaging yourself. If you suspect that you are depressed, see your doctor about this common problem, which often comes from unrelenting stress. You may find that your other problems are easier to solve once your depression has been treated appropriately. Incidentally, having a healthy diet and exercising regularly is a recognized part of the treatment of common forms of depression.

Reinforcing your habits is not something you do just once. It is an ongoing process that moves you to new and better goals throughout your life. Losing weight is just the first step in improving your inner health. To continue to reinforce your diet you will need some inspiration. One of the most effective means of inspiring people to change is to tell them real-life stories of others who changed their lives, and in Step 5 you will learn about how to inspire yourself to be successful.

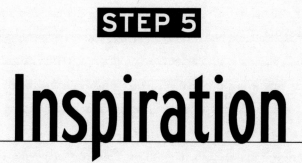

STEP 5

Inspiration

Finding Your Inner Voice and Vision

Now you have all the tools you need to change. You have the nutritional, practical, and behavioral knowledge you need to change your life, and if you've started to implement the program, you may already be starting to notice some positive changes. You even have some tools to help you keep your new behaviors intact. This chapter is about finding the inner strength to make this new life your own.

I want you to own your weight loss. This won't happen overnight. In my clinical programs, I tell patients that they don't own their new weight loss until they have kept the weight off for six months to a year.

In this secular era, I have to be careful what I say about religion. Religion has been blamed for the Middle East crisis, terrorism, and wars throughout history. However, when you peel away the organizations around religion, what you find at the core of all religions and forms of spirituality is the search for an inner voice.

Most of us go through the day without giving much thought to spirituality. In fact, most of us don't slow down enough to be able to hear our inner voice. There are many examples of the power of the inner voice, which scientists call mind-body interaction. In traditional Chinese medicine, there is the practice of Qi Gong (pronounced chee-gong). In this exercise, you learn to slow down a few minutes each day and get in touch with yourself. One of my professors at Harvard Medical School, Dr. Herbert Benson, wrote a book many years ago called *The Relaxation Response*. He was able to use Western science to demonstrate that the mind could affect the body's blood pressure, temperature, and breathing. You may have seen the mimes who stand on street corners hours on end in the same position, with very shallow breathing. They achieve this state through deep meditation.

Patients sometimes tell me they eat different types of Trigger Foods depending on their emotional state. If they are angry, they want salty foods. If they are sad, they want sweet foods or chocolate. Meditation during the day as a separate activity or active rethinking of problems while you exercise can reduce your overall stress level and the need for Trigger Foods.

Stress and the Relaxation Response

You can lower your blood pressure, pulse, and body temperature by relaxing. Even your brain waves are different when you are relaxed. They are not as slow as when you are sleeping, but they are not in the state of high alert that many people carry around with them while commuting or sitting at their desk at work.

As I go through my day, I see lots of people who are not relaxed. Their faces are flushed as they raise their voices and speak quickly, interrupting others before they can get through a sentence. Their pulses race and their breathing is shallow. This type of behavior, sometimes called type A, can be the result of high levels of stress hormones. These hormones, called "catecholamines," come from the adrenal gland. Their levels go up with stress to levels ten to one hundred times normal and raise blood pressure, pulse, and body temperature. For people with high blood pressure, this is often the trigger to a stroke.

It is important to differentiate this destructive type A behavior, which is turned inward, from high-energy behavior, which is expressed outwardly without the inner stress and anger characteristic of type A behavior. Scientists have found that the classic rapid-fire type A personality is associated with a fight-or-flight response in most individuals who behave this way.

Stress comes in many flavors, and some people are able to control stress so that they look relaxed on the outside (such as a professional golfer making a $50,000 putt), but on the inside they are a bundle of nerves. This is the worst kind of stress and can lead to diseases and conditions that are not obviously related to stress, including heartburn, irritable bowel syndrome (constipation and/or frequent bowel movements), eruptions of acne, bladder pain, frequent urination, muscle aches, and back pain.

Since weight gain is also a stress-related disorder, many of these health problems often come along with it. I have seen thousands of patients suffering from both overweight and one of these other conditions. In fact, one year I saw so many patients with overweight in combination with lower back pain and knee pain that an insurance company reviewing my medical records listed me in their directory under the specialty of physical medicine instead of nutrition.

The symptoms of stress-related disorders aren't necessarily attached in an obvious way to their original cause. But you need to know the cause in order to solve the problem, or you'll run into trouble. Many of the most popular drugs attempt (often unsuccessfully) to treat problems such as migraine headaches associated with overweight that disappear once the stress is relieved or controlled.

While you often cannot control the job or family situation causing your stress, you can find ways to control your reaction to it. For example, you can remove yourself physically from the source of the stress. You can take a break from the stress. You can plan on how to reduce or resolve the stressing events. You can substitute a healthy for an unhealthy behavior in reacting to the stress. You can reorganize your office, your desk, your bedroom, or your calendar to reduce your stress. You can add meditation to your life as a separate habit or as part of your exercise routine (discussed in the next chapter) to help reduce your stress. As you balance yourself physically, emotionally, intellectually, and spiritually, you will find that you are reacting less to the same stressful events. I will give you examples of how individuals faced with the same stresses changed their responses so that they did not set up the vicious cycle of stress eating.

Listening to Your Inner Voice While You Meditate

Meditation is the process of slowing down enough to experience the present. I have a good friend who likes to say, "The past is history, the future is a mystery, but today is a gift. That is why they call it the present." So few of us live in the here and now. We are worried about when we will get to our next destination or what we could have done in the past to make something come out differently. Even if you could have acted differently in the past to avoid a bad result, it won't help to dwell on it now and ruin the present.

To meditate, set aside at least 5 minutes in your home or office to breathe and relax. Make sure you can't be disturbed. Lie down flat on the floor with a pillow under your head and close your eyes. Count to three as you inhale and count to four as you exhale. Think only about your breathing. When you are feeling relaxed and about to finish your breathing break, slowly open your eyes and resume your normal breathing pattern. When you feel comfortable meditating for 5 minutes, extend your meditation to

15 minutes. Soon you may find that this time is so pleasant that you enjoy a full 30 minutes of meditation.

As you breathe, you may find it hard to keep your mind focused on your breathing. If this happens, you can focus on a word, an image, or a sound. You can pick an object in the room or hang a mobile in the air that you use for your focus point. You can put on a favorite relaxing piece of music that enables you to relax or even a background sound, such as that of a river, the ocean, or the wind. You can also repeat a word to yourself that is meaningful and enables you to center your thoughts.

If meditating in stillness is impossible for you, then you can stretch or do yoga while you meditate. If your muscles cramp up while you meditate, you may not be relaxed fully. Try to think about your muscle groups and be sure they are relaxed. Stretching against a wall or chair or simply assuming yoga positions can reduce stress by relieving the cramping sensation in your muscles and joints.

Sitting at your desk or computer tenses up the muscles of the neck, upper back, shoulders, and chest. Stand up every 30 minutes and stretch your neck muscles by rotating your head slowly. Then shrug your shoulders. Stretch your arms out in front of you and move your arms forward and backward in small circles. Then hold your fists in front of your eyes and move them outward, as if you were holding dumbbells, and move them to your sides until your elbows move back and slightly behind your back. You should feel a warm stretch in the middle of your chest. Do this and all stretches slowly to get the full benefit.

To stretch your lower back, lie down flat on the floor. With your left leg extended straight, bend your right leg and put your right foot flat on the floor. Now slowly lift your left leg until it is about halfway up. You should feel a gentle stretch in your lower back. Do this five to ten times, and then reverse positions so that you raise your right leg with your left leg bent. Now lie on your right side and raise your left leg while keeping your right leg bent. (Lie on a pillow if it is more comfortable.) Switch legs.

You have now mastered the art of stretching and relaxation, so it is possible to go on to listening to your inner voice in other situations, including the time you spend each day doing exercise.

Listening to Your Inner Voice While You Exercise

In the next chapter, you'll learn about the *L.A. Shape Diet* exercise plan, but I find that an important part of exercise is active meditation. Read on and learn how following your inner voice can make exercising more satisfying, fun, and relaxing.

I am not bored by exercise. I don't need to watch television or listen to talk radio while exercising. When I exercise, I listen to calm music as I allow my mind to wander and work out things that are nagging at me. My mind contemplates, reduces worry, and finds solutions to problems while I am exercising. Most problems don't seem so big once they have been mulled over.

Focusing on the movements you make during exercise reduces your stress levels. By focusing on your exercise movements, you will distract your mind from what is stressing you. As you will see, exercise is the only healthy addiction. When you finish exercising, as when you finish meditating, you will feel refreshed and restored in mind, body, and soul.

Meditation Leads to Inspiration

Besides refreshing you and reducing stress, meditation can lead to inspiration. This happens almost magically. You are thinking about something, or even nothing at all, and suddenly you have an insight. I don't know where insights come from or how the brain consciously develops new ones. Religious people believe all inspiration comes from God, while secularists believe it is a physiological brain function. In fact, modern brain scans using positron emission tomography (PET) have shown that areas of the brain associated with vision light up during dreaming. So it may be the combination of activities in different brain areas that leads to new insights.

In ancient times, philosophers contemplated the origin of the universe and claimed to have dreams and visions of God that revealed to them how the universe started. Mystical systems such as Kabbalah in Judaism, revelations in Ecstatic Christianity, and Zen Buddhism are based on the power of contemplation to bring about visions and insights, and they are often credited with being able to predict the future. You can discover a whole new side of yourself by allowing your mind to quiet down and explore your present reality. Creativity cannot enter into a cluttered, multitasking mind. Albert Einstein was perhaps the most creative mind of recent centuries. He was famous for saying, "God does not play dice with the universe." He believed his laws were not simply right by chance due to the workings of probability theory. He believed that somehow his insights about time and space were inspired thoughts. What is amazing is that he was proven right again and again. With every new telescope mounted in space comes more proof that Einstein was right. How else can one explain Leonardo da Vinci's vision of the helicopter, or Jules Verne's visions of submarines long before they existed?

It is possible that inspiration is just another wonderful manifestation of human brain function. The ability to imagine what will be and invent new things is a great power. I want you to use this awesome power to strengthen your inner nature to seek and maintain good health for life. Your vision of where and why you want to lose weight and keep it off is personal. In this chapter, I'll share success stories drawn from the thousands of stories I have heard, so that you may find some things to inspire you to lose weight and seek optimum nutritional health. Magic doesn't happen, and the basis for your changes is scientific. It is the inspiration that will make these changes happen according to the scientific laws that regulate your body. In other words, you can't think your way thin.

Science for Success

Inspiration is a tool that can help you achieve your goals in combination with diet, exercise, and behavioral change. It is a very powerful tool, but it cannot work by itself. There must still be science behind your success, and there is.

Thousands of people just like you have lost weight and kept it off with a program of meal replacements, adequate protein, and lots of fruits and vegetables described in this book as part of a healthy overall diet and lifestyle. I have studied hundreds of people in formal scientific studies, and seen thousands of patients in my clinical practice who have succeeded. I have traveled internationally and heard the testimonial of individuals in dozens of languages as they describe their weight loss and how it changed their lives.

Weight gain can occur for many different reasons. For example, I have seen patients who gained weight eating huge amounts of food after a divorce or the loss of a job. These people were going to become fat whether they ate healthy food or not. They were using food as a drug to reduce stress, but it was not working. Only by rediscovering themselves were they able to move beyond these life-changing events and stop overeating.

Of course, individual rates of weight loss on any program will vary. The biggest reason for this variation beyond the physical differences that determine the rate of weight loss is the personal investment of individuals in their own success. As that great twentieth-century philosopher Yogi Berra said, "If people don't want to come to the ballpark, there is nothing you can do to stop them!"

In my clinical work, I have often seen a mother try to convince her daughter to lose weight without success, only to have the daughter return on her own after several years and succeed with the same diet. On the first visit, the weight loss was for her mother, and it didn't happen. When she returned, she reminded me of the first visit and told me that it would be different this time. This time she was losing weight for herself and not her mother.

Science is important in explaining how much weight you can realistically lose if you follow this program carefully. However, there is no amount of science that will guarantee your success. Only you can guarantee your success by following through on your plans to lose weight and keep it off.

Success Stories

Knowing that others have succeeded can help you visualize your own success. The stories that follow, which are adapted from real-life cases in my office, emphasize how weight loss changed these people's lives. In the interest of patient confidentiality, I have disguised the identities, and any resemblance to real individuals is purely coincidental.

These stories are not unusual. In fact, I had so many similar stories that I had to choose among them for this chapter. What all of them have in common is a key moment of decision and action. All the positive results these people experienced flowed from this single moment. In each case, the motivating factor was different. In some cases, a painful injury triggered weight gain, and more pain led to action. In other cases, it was the desire to reach a specific goal for a special occasion that made the difference. What will it be for you?

MAN IN HIS MID-FORTIES

I was a lousy eater. I would skip breakfast and have a coffee latté on my way to work. By 11 A.M., I was feeling hunger pangs, and would go looking for the doughnut cart. Lunch was always on the run at a fast-food joint near my work. By the late afternoon, I would be hungry again and stop in at a fast-food place for some fries on the way home. My wife always made really healthy dinners and couldn't figure out why I was gaining weight.

After I started the L.A. Shape program, I would have a shake for breakfast and feel full until noon. At lunch, I would have another shake, and I'd eat a protein bar in the car on the way home. By the time I got started on dinner, I felt much more in control. In the last six weeks I lost twenty-five pounds and feel stronger and more energetic. This is the first diet I've been on that makes me feel full of energy—and I am finally free of those hunger pangs.

WOMAN IN HER THIRTIES

I was a size 8 until I got pregnant. I gained 40 pounds and three dress sizes with my pregnancy, and never really lost that weight. I just hated the way I looked, and I didn't feel sexy at all. It was hectic enough to have to get up in the middle of the night, and I was miserable thinking that this would be the way I would look. I really didn't want to turn into my mother.

The shakes on the L.A. Shape Diet were really delicious, and I was able to make them in the kitchen in my blender while I prepared my baby's food. I felt full and satisfied with my shakes at breakfast and lunch. I am finally beginning to take off some of my weight. I lost 10 pounds in the first four weeks, and I'm on my way to losing all my extra weight. I am joining a Mommy and Me exercise group to help bring some movement back into my daily routine and I feel positive again about getting back to my old dress size.

WOMAN IN HER EARLY FIFTIES

I've always thought of myself as healthy, but since I turned fifty I have noticed this awful spare tire on my stomach. I have no idea how it happened. I thought I was eating the same amount, but I still gained weight. I tried starving myself, but I couldn't seem to make any progress at all.

Once I started my shakes at breakfast and lunch I had more energy. It was so much better than trying to starve and eat mini-portions of my favorite foods. I started walking every day, and I am finally losing weight for the first time. I have more energy, and I am thrilled to have lost 8 pounds in three weeks. My waistline is smaller, and my clothes feel looser.

MAN IN HIS TWENTIES

I've been fat all my life. Kids made fun of me, starting in kindergarten. My mother took me to lots of doctors, but nothing worked. I got a great job as a computer technician, but no women looked my way.

The day I started this plan, my life was changed. I found out that I was burning a lot of calories every day, and that I could eat a lot more than I thought and still could lose up to 12 pounds per month. Now, five months into the program, I have lost 60 pounds, and I don't have as far to go as I thought. I learned that my target weight was higher than I realized. This is also the first diet on which I don't feel hungry. I am eating more healthy protein than I ever did before, and I have the energy to lift weights at the gym.

I was always strong underneath, but now my muscles are showing. I met a nice girl at the gym, and I think things are going to be a lot better for me now that I found the answers.

WOMAN IN HER TWENTIES

I was really skinny until I became a teenager. At about age thirteen, I blossomed out all over. I started getting fat and never stopped. I didn't have a clue as to why I was gaining weight. My mom took me to see a specialist, and he gave me thyroid pills, but they didn't help. I just got fatter. It was no fun. I was home alone all the time on the weekends, and no one asked me to my high school prom.

I now work as a secretary and sit around all day. About six months ago, I started on this new plan on which I drink shakes for breakfast and lunch with extra protein. I have lost over 30 pounds, and I am wearing some great new clothes. People at the office have been giving me compliments about my new figure. This is the best I have felt in years. I have more energy to get through the day, and I feel great about myself and my new body.

MAN IN HIS THIRTIES

I'm a salesman, and I sit around all day in my car. I drive from one town to another for days. All the food on the road is full of fat, and eating is the only thing that really breaks up the boredom of my days. In just one year I gained over 50 pounds. That's a lot of blue plate specials.

Once I discovered this plan, I felt that I was finally able to control myself. Don't get me wrong—I still go out for a good meal once in a while. But every day I have a shake for breakfast and a shake for lunch. Then I'm careful about what I order for dinner. One great thing I learned is that I need a lot more protein than I ever thought I did. I eat 6 ounces of lean meat at dinner, and I put more than 25 grams of protein in my shakes at breakfast and lunch. It's a lot easier than I thought. I keep a shaker with me and shake up my drinks every morning and at lunch with some nonfat milk. I eat protein bars when I am in the car as an afternoon snack. I'm not hungry between meals at all, and I have already lost about 26 pounds in just eight weeks. My back used to hurt from sitting in the car all day, and now it feels just great. I feel more confident now, and my sales numbers are up.

MAN IN HIS SIXTIES

I thought life was going to be fun when I retired. I didn't count on all the hours I would have on my hands. When I first retired, I wore a path in my carpet from the living room to the kitchen. The refrigerator door would open and close every time there was a commercial on television, and I got bored. I was watching more than thirty hours a week of television. Then I remembered that I had some golf clubs in the basement that I got as a gift from my boss. I hadn't touched them in years. So I picked up my clubs and went to the range. As I tried to look down at the golf ball, I was shocked to realize I could barely see over my stomach without bending forward. This was not going to work. I started on a high-protein shake for breakfast, made with berries in a blender right in my kitchen. Boy, it tastes great. I feel full of energy and am not hungry at all. Then I take off for the golf course. I practice for a couple of hours and go home and make another shake. Right after lunch I go back to play eighteen holes. I have a protein bar at the turn. By the time I get home, I am ready for dinner, but I'm not as ravenous as I used to be. Now I eat dinner more slowly and enjoy it. I have lost more than 20 pounds in just six weeks, and I'm starting to hit the ball pretty straight now that I can see where it is.

WOMAN IN HER SEVENTIES

I have always been pretty careful about what I eat, but after my husband passed away last year, I was hungry all the time. I grew this beach ball around the area below my waist, and I couldn't fit into any of my clothes. My greatest joy is playing with my grandchildren, but I tried to skip meals to lose weight and all that happened was that my energy level got really low.

I started on these great-tasting shakes that fill you up. I have one for breakfast and one for lunch. If I meet my girlfriends for lunch, I will have my shake beforehand and order a salad with nonfat dressing and a glass of iced tea so I have something to do while we are all talking together.

I actually lost 10 pounds in the last month, and that beach ball on my stomach is starting to get smaller. I went to see my doctor, and he told me that he was really happy I was losing weight. My blood pressure was better and my cholesterol levels had gone down, all due to my losing weight. I really feel great about my new way of life.

Writing Your Success Story

Now it's time to write down your own vision of where you want to be. I always say to my patients, "Begin with the end in mind." You know about your lean body mass and target weight, but what is your personal goal for the weight you want to lose in the next three months, six months, and one year? You may revise this later, but it is important to know your personal goals.

Inspiration

How Losing Weight and Getting Fit Can Change Your Life

Nearly everyone who loses weight notices some big changes in their lives. Not only do their bodies feel better, but they are perceived differently by their family, friends, colleagues, and employers. They appear more confident and have a better quality of life. Here are some of the ways in which people's lives have been changed through weight loss:

1   Met the girl (guy) of my dreams.

2   Got a promotion at work.

3   Went to the beach with my kids and felt good about my body.

4   Fit into some great clothes I bought years ago.

5   Got lots of compliments and felt more confident with friends.

6   Bought some new clothes I would never have considered when I was heavy.

7   Took up a new sport (bicycling, weight lifting, golf, tennis).

8   My sleep improved, and I wake up more rested.

9   I stopped taking medication for my cholesterol and high blood pressure.

10   My knees and back don't hurt as much anymore.

11   My asthma improved, so I have fewer and less severe attacks.

12   I feel positive about each day and I don't get blue so often.

How will your life change?

1   _____

2   _____

3   _____

4   _____

5   _____

Every Day Is a New Opportunity

As you visualize your success, start each new day as if it were your first day on the program. Don't take your progress for granted as you move toward your goal. Write down your weight every week and keep a chart of your progress. You should see a steady downward trend. One way to stay motivated is to look at your personal vision of success every day and make sure you don't waste the opportunity to make progress toward your goal whenever possible.

Reward Yourself for Maintaining Your Momentum

Whenever you have reached a weekly goal weight, note it in your journal and give yourself a reward. Some of my patients put marbles in a jar and buy themselves a gift when the jar is full of marbles. This should be an ongoing process for the rest of your life as you keep rewarding yourself for your progress. But be sure to give yourself nonfood rewards, such as a new pair of shoes or a gadget you've had your eye on. If you like to buy fitness equipment, so much the better as you get ready for the next chapter.

Exercise for Life

Doing nothing is more appealing than doing something—especially when you are as stressed out as most Americans are today. Perhaps that explains why 24 percent of all Americans never exercise and another 25 percent don't exercise regularly.

This lack of activity is a major factor in the modern epidemic of obesity as our work and home lives have become easier physically because of labor-saving devices such as remote controls and garage door openers. Most of us drive everywhere, and the assembly line jobs of yesteryear requiring heavy physical labor have largely disappeared as the manufacturing sector in this country has shrunk. Now we are an information-based society, and most people work in service industries where they are behind the counter, driving a car or truck, or sitting in front of a computer all day. Many more women are in the workforce and have to hold down a job and care for their families. The two-income family has left about 15 minutes for preparing dinner, and you have no time for exercise unless you program it into your life.

In this chapter, I am going to start slow, just get you active at first, then I will take you through the steps to building muscle with some great exercises that my successful patients do regularly. If you are already active, skip ahead to the formal information on exercise training. Otherwise, start slowly and get hooked on what I call the only healthy addiction—regular exercise.

Get Moving

Millions of American men and women get out of bed, take their morning shower, get in their car, sit at their desk all day, sit in their cars as they commute home, eat dinner, and then fall asleep after eating snacks in front of the TV all evening. Millions more stay at home with small children, exert a little energy running errands in the car, feed the kids and husband in the evening, and collapse in front of the TV as they finish off the day eating snacks. You know these people. If the urge to exercise happens to come over them, they wait until it passes. Is this you?

Breaking the Barriers

What are the barriers between you and a regular exercise program?

1. "I don't have the time." Time passes at different rates. If you are waiting in the doctor's office for an extra hour, time passes slowly. If you are enjoying a last day of vacation, time seems to rush by. I'm asking you to make some time to get moving and to exercise.

Even though you may think you do not have the time right now, you can make the time by cutting out wasted moments somewhere else in your life. A lot of time is wasted watching television. I can't understand why people can't find time to exercise when many watch two or three hours of television every night.

Take a hard look at your life, starting with the weekends. Can you find a few hours on a Saturday or Sunday to go for a walk in the park by yourself, with a family member or friend, or with a pet? This can be the first step you take to get moving. You will find this time so relaxing that you'll extend it to one or two days a week—and then you're on your way toward a daily walking and weight-lifting routine.

2. "My muscles always hurt when I exercise, and I get short of breath." If you're out of shape, you have to ease into your exercise routine by dressing warmly and stretching properly beforehand. I stretch throughout the day to reduce stress, especially the small muscles around my neck and shoulders.

If you have injured your muscles before in an exercise program, you should avoid lifting more weight than you can comfortably handle. I remember going to the gym once and assuming I could begin with barbell curls with 20-pound weights after not having exercised for more than a year. The next day, my muscles hurt so much I could barely move my arms.

In this chapter, you'll learn how to build your muscle by creating a gentle burning rather than a pain in your muscles after each weight-lifting exercise. You'll learn how to keep the amount of weight you lift in any exercise under control by using special movements and paying attention to proper form and posture in doing each movement. The idea of "no pain, no gain" is dangerous and out of fashion.

If you've been short of breath while running track in high school, you remember it as an unpleasant experience. Your brain tells your diaphragm to breathe harder to get rid of the carbon dioxide in your lungs and bring in more oxygen. It hurts because the diaphragm, a sheetlike muscle at the base of the lungs, has pain fibers like any other muscle. You won't be feeling that kind of discomfort on this exercise plan because you won't be doing that type of exercise. You'll learn to use walking, a treadmill, or elliptical exercise machine at a heart rate that burns fat but does not leave you breathless. In fact, at the proper heart rate, you should be able to carry on a conversation.

3. "Exercise is boring." Going to the gym can be a break from your routine. Some gyms are even open 24 hours, so you can pick a time that fits your schedule. Take a shower at the gym and relax on the weekends, or get in and out quickly for a compact workout during the week—the choice is yours. If you want to exercise at home, create a special space that you set up as your home gym. This can be a corner of your house or apartment where you leave your gym equipment. You may already have some equipment that you use mainly to hold your clothing. You spent the money on it, so you may as well use it!

Choose a well-lit area, if you can, and set up a small radio or CD player so you can listen to some music while you exercise. If you go to a gym, bring a headset with you. Create a total environment, including comfortable light and music that will inspire you, and have an energy bar and water bottle with you while you work out. If you get hungry during a late-afternoon workout, eating a protein bar can help you finish your workout in good form so that you avoid a muscle strain.

You have to get into the exercise lifestyle. Read fitness magazines and books and buy new clothes for working out. Get back to your college days with some logo wear from your favorite university, or buy workout T-shirts on vacation that will remind you of your special place to get away. As you get into this experience, you won't find it boring—you'll get the pleasant rush you feel from doing a favorite activity.

Aerobic and Heavy Resistance Exercise

Exercise is generally divided into two categories: aerobic exercise and heavy resistance exercise (which usually takes the form of weight lifting). This division is a little artificial, since almost all exercises raise both your heart rate and exercise some muscles. However, it is useful to devote part of any formal workout sessions you schedule to these two classes of exercise.

Exercising Your Heart Muscle: Aerobics

Aerobics is the scientific term for getting your heart rate increased enough to exercise your heart muscle. In ancient times, humans had no choice but to expend energy in aerobic exercise. If there was a saber-toothed tiger after you, it was time to start running. Today we have to make an appointment with ourselves for walking, running, or other forms of aerobic exercise.

Aerobic exercise requires large muscle movements over a sustained period of time, delivering oxygen to the cardiovascular system and elevating your heart rate to at least 50 percent of your maximum heart rate for a period of 20 minutes. Take a moment to calculate your personal target heart rate (THR) now:

220 MINUS YOUR AGE = MAXIMUM HEART RATE (MHR)

(MHR—Resting Heart Rate) × 0.5 + Resting Heart Rate = THR 50

(MHR—Resting Heart Rate) × 0.6 + Resting Heart Rate = THR 60

(MHR—Resting Heart Rate) × 0.7 + Resting Heart Rate = THR 70

(The special math for the THR 50, THR 60, and THR 70 account for different resting heart rates among individuals at different levels of conditioning. Some gyms simplify this calculation by simply taking a percentage of your age-adjusted maximum heart rate. These targets are just a guide for you to understand how to exercise in a safe range of heart rates. So don't get carried away with exact calculations.)

To measure your Resting Heart Rate sit quietly for 15 minutes and take your pulse for ten seconds and multiply by six.

First week: Exercise at about THR 50 for 20 minutes.

Weeks 2 to 12: Exercise at about THR 60 for 30 minutes.

In good condition: Exercise at about THR 70 for 30 minutes.

Target heart rates are not single numbers, but represent an acceptable range from 50 to 80 percent of your age-adjusted Maximum Heart Rate. You can get adequate heart muscle protection from the lower ranges above. It has been proven that you will burn more fat if you can exercise a longer time at a lower heart rate than if you exhaust yourself at a higher heart rate for a shorter period of time. So pick a rate at which you get a comfortable degree of exercise and feel warm and sweaty toward the end of your aerobic workout. At the right heart rate, aerobic exercise should be something pleasant that you want to do again. Don't rush the difficulty of the exercise. You should follow the scale on page 170 gradually as your fitness improves:

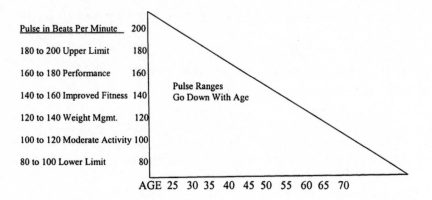

Pulse in Beats Per Minute   200

180 to 200 Upper Limit   180

160 to 180 Performance   160

140 to 160 Improved Fitness 140   Pulse Ranges
                                        Go Down With Age
120 to 140 Weight Mgmt.   120

100 to 120 Moderate Activity 100

80 to 100 Lower Limit   80

AGE 25 30 35 40 45 50 55 60 65 70

TAKE AEROBIC EXERCISE TO THE NEXT LEVEL

For years most government agencies and academics like me recommended at least three aerobic sessions of 20 minutes or more each week to condition the heart and at least four sessions of 45 minutes of heavy resistance activity such as weight lifting each week for long-term weight loss. The National Academy of Sciences has since increased its recommendation to 30 to 60 minutes of aerobic exercise a day. The reaction to this increase in recommended exercise was surprise and skepticism. How could you ask a population that was not attaining your current recommendation to exercise even more? Other experts, including Dr. Jim Hill of the University of Colorado, argued that minimal levels of exercise, such as a few thousand steps a day, when combined with a very small reduction in food intake comparable to a small handful of candy (100 calories) could solve the problem of obesity by reducing the constant weight gain in our society. While getting moving is a great start, as I suggested earlier, I would like to encourage you to take your exercise to the next level to make a difference in your shape—the L.A. Shape way!

If you set the ultimate goal of 1 hour per day of exercise, you may ultimately surprise yourself and attain your goal. Exercise shouldn't be a struggle, but if you want to be lean and healthy, you have to work for it.

Choose an activity you enjoy so that it will be easier to incorporate it into your daily life, and you will experience the physiological, psychological, and biochemical benefits of exercise. Supplement your workouts with active recreational activities that you enjoy.

FITTING IN AEROBIC ACTIVITY

Among the easiest ways to increase your calorie-burning activities are: Walking upstairs instead of taking an elevator anytime you go up three or fewer stories. Walking after dinner can help digestion and mood while it burns up calories.

The first step to getting more active is simply to get moving. Wear comfortable walking shoes and get out with your family, friends, or neighbors for a morning or evening walk. If this is impractical, walk at lunch after you have had your Empowering Shake. Giving yourself permission to change and powering through the first week is the key to starting a lifelong habit. Walking is the first step to getting going, and it is easy to do during lunch or at anytime you have 15 to 30 minutes. Or break up the walk into several sessions that add up to 30 minutes.

You can also choose fun activities, such as gardening or golf, or others, like cleaning the yard, raking leaves, and planting trees. Schedule these activities every weekend to keep your bones and muscles working.

On the following page are some examples of exercises that can be used toward fulfilling your daily total aerobic exercise. The list includes both less vigorous activities that take more time and moves, and those that are more vigorous and take less time.

So, just pick an activity you like and go to it. However, you need to make it a regular habit. I personally like doing formal exercise sessions at a gym or at home and counting the activities listed here as a bonus to burn more fat.

Fitness Around the House or at Play

Household activities

Washing and waxing a car for 45 to 60 minutes

Washing windows or mopping for 45 to 60 minutes

Pushing a stroller 2 miles in 40 minutes

Raking leaves for 45 to 60 minutes

Gardening for 30 to 45 minutes

Walking in the mall to and from a store for 40 minutes

Similar household chore of your choice for 30 to 45 minutes

Sports and leisure activities

Playing volleyball for 45 minutes

Playing touch football for 30 to 45 minutes

Shooting baskets for 30 minutes

Similar sports activity of your choice for 30 minutes

Bicycling 5 miles in 30 minutes

Dancing fast for 30 minutes

Jog-walking 2 miles in 30 minutes

Doing water aerobics for 30 minutes

Swimming laps for 20 minutes

Along with your daily exercise, experts recommend that you take 10,000 steps a day. A pedometer is a great way to keep track of how many steps you take in the course of a day. These devices register a step whenever your body moves up and down. It is also a good idea to wear one all day for at least a few days to see that you are really increasing your activities overall. Some studies show that after exercising for 30 minutes on a treadmill or bicycle, you may go easy on yourself and skip walking the dog, or you may just flop down on the couch. As a result, your overall activity for the day may be the same as before you started your formal exercise program, and your dog won't be too thrilled, either. It will only help to burn fat faster if you do more activities in addition to your regular workout to keep your heart healthy.

Start by stretching before you exercise. Stretching helps to keep your muscles from getting hurt during even gentle aerobic exercise. If you don't know how to stretch, get a book on stretching or ask a fitness instructor to help you customize some stretches. Then get on a treadmill or bicycle or elliptical trainer and warm up for 10 minutes, going progressively faster until you achieve your personal target heart rate, which you calculated using the table on page 169. I like to use the elliptical trainer at the gym, since it puts less stress than a treadmill on my knees, hips, and back.

If you are into gadgets, you can buy a pulse meter, which you wear as a watch along with a chest strap that senses the electrical impulses in your heart. Many of the elliptical trainers, treadmills, and bicycles in gyms have pulse sensors that you activate by holding on to a metal grip. Also, remember that you should be able to hold a conversation comfortably the entire time you're exercising.

After 20 minutes at about your personal target heart rate, start your cool-down by walking more slowly. If you're on an automatic treadmill or stationary bicycle, it can be programmed to provide you with a gradual cool-down.

Heavy Resistance Exercise: Why Lift Weights?

Weight lifting is the second pillar of your exercise routine and is critical to your efforts to raise metabolism through exercise. If you lift weights with a short period of rest between exercises, you build up a pretty good sweat and get your heart beating in the process so you get some aerobic benefit, too.

However, the primary purpose of weight lifting is to build muscle. Since a pound of muscle burns 14 calories per day at rest, building muscle is the best way to raise your metabolism (the amount of calories you burn). Just a 10-pound increase in muscle means that you can burn another 140 calories per day at rest. That means you can lose $\frac{1}{3}$ pound more per week eating the same amount of food, or you can eat an additional 140 calories per day, or almost 1,000 calories per week, and still maintain your weight once you reach your target weight. Also, when you are doing either aerobics or weight lifting you are not eating, which means you are practicing the best exercise for weight loss: walking away from the refrigerator door.

BUILDING MUSCLE

When you lift weights, you help your health by building muscle cells. During the stretching part of the muscle action (on a biceps curl, this would be when you move your arm down), your muscles fatigue and then get a very slight inflammation. The signals from this purposeful inflammation are the same as those given off by an infection or tumor, but in this case the signals recruit new baby muscle cells, called "satellite myocytes," which merge with the damaged muscle fiber to enlarge it. Some oxidation accompanying the inflammation of the muscle cells is inevitable, but the resulting cell damage can be minimized by eating protein after you exercise. It is also important to eat a diet rich in the antioxidants found in fruits and vegetables to minimize the damage to your muscles. Some studies have shown that taking vitamin E at a dose of 200 IU or more in the days before exercising can do the same thing.

Why bother building your muscles if you are going to damage them in the process? It was shown in studies done in 1948 that weight-bearing exercises were the best way to rebuild muscles in military personnel who were trying to build muscle after knee surgery. The details on this background science and how to optimize your weight-lifting routine using the latest breakthroughs in exercise science and physiology can be found in the Appendix (pages 281–297). For now, I want to get you started with a simple and easily understood regimen, because studies show that over the first twelve weeks these standard exercises get the same great results in untrained individuals as the most complex weight-lifting routines. After three months, you may want to refer to the Appendix and to fitness magazines to learn more advanced techniques.

Weight-bearing exercise is essential to maintaining the strength of your bones, your posture, and your ability to achieve and keep a healthy body weight. By building muscle you become more efficient at burning calories, and so you have more leeway in your diet as you retain a healthy body weight.

GETTING STARTED WITH WEIGHT LIFTING

Circuit training is weight training in which you move from one exercise to another with little rest in between. Going faster and using lighter weights can improve heart health and endurance, while going slower and using heavier weights can build strength and muscle size, speeding up metabolism. You need to spend more time between groups of repetitions (called sets) if you lift heavier weights.

It is definitely true that doing lighter exercises and more repetitions will avoid building bulky muscles, which is often the preference of women. So, if you want the strength without the bulk, do more repetitions at lighter weights (see the Appendix for more details).

You can turn any workout into a circuit by going from one exercise to the next, with no more than a 15- to 30-second rest period. Repeat the circuit three times in about 30 minutes for maximum benefit. You should focus on one set of muscles one day and another on another day so that the same muscle groups get a chance to recover before the next bout of exercise.

Your Exercise Routine: A Three-Day Cycle

Day 1: chest and triceps exercises (similar muscle groups)
Day 2: back and biceps exercises (similar muscle groups)
Day 3: shoulder and leg exercises (what's left–not similar muscle groups)

You could repeat this cycle twice and have one rest day per week in between, but choose to go in a continuous cycle. One day off is never a tragedy, but try not to let a string of days go by without a workout. Your goal is to make your circuit training a habit.

While circuit training may sound like a lot of exercise to be done in a short amount of time, it's still important to concentrate on every movement you make, especially when you are lowering the weight.

This second movement is when your weaker muscles usually come into play—you're stretching both the stronger (agonist) and weaker (antagonist) muscles. For example, when you do a biceps curl, the biceps work more on the way up and the triceps on the way down. The biceps' muscle fibers are overstretched at the very end of this movement, which is called an eccentric movement. While all movements during a weight-lifting exercise should be done slowly and with control, it is particularly important to make the eccentric move slowly. It is at this point of overstretching muscle fibers that the key signals are sent to the muscle cells to increase their size. So count two seconds up and four seconds down on a biceps curl.

The key to building muscle is to feel a burning in your biceps after about 10 repetitions and to continue carefully to between 12 and 15 repetitions. Your triceps are important because they balance the weight, and if you move too quickly you can injure your ligaments.

I used the biceps and triceps as an example because most people are familiar with those muscles. However, think of any large joint and imagine which is the dominant and which the nondominant muscle at the joint. If the joint is envisioned as a pulley, then the unbalanced stress at the joint will cause the pulley wheel to wear. The same thing happens with your joints over long periods of time. So, when you're lifting weights, you make sure both sets of muscles are being built up in a balanced fashion.

As you do each exercise, stay focused on the movement and maintain your balance. If you feel out of control, reduce the weight to a level that allows you to do the exercise correctly. An injury will cause inflammation that will damage your muscle even more, and pain from injuries to ligaments and joints can permanently sideline you not only from weight lifting but also from life. As I said earlier, the old adage "no pain, no gain" is simply not true.

How do people usually overdo an exercise? The mind can lift what the body cannot. In your rush to build up muscle, you may be adding too much weight too soon. The general rule is that if you can do an extra repetition easily, go ahead and do it. Then, at the next exercise session in which you do the same movement, add another 10 percent to the weight you are lifting at the same number of repetitions. Injuries usually happen when you lift almost as much as you can for a few repetitions, then do another repetition with very bad form so that your joints go out of alignment. Your weaker muscle is injured as it tries to rebalance the weight.

If you overdo the exercise, rest for a few days until you are ready to resume your routine without pain. While you are healing, use a nonsteroidal

Exercise for Life

anti-inflammatory drug, such as ibuprofen, Naprosyn, or aspirin, to relieve your aches and pains. Use ice packs on damaged joints to reduce inflammation until you are comfortable in a normal range of motion. If your pain is really severe or doesn't respond to usual pain relievers, you had better see a doctor. You may have a tendinitis that will respond to physical therapy, or you may have damaged one of your joints.

COMMON WEIGHT-LIFTING EXERCISES

There are many different exercise routines you can use effectively, depending upon the equipment you have available. The descriptions below are not exhaustive, and you can find a lot more ideas in fitness magazines and books. Some of the exercises below require gym equipment, but I've tried to provide an alternative exercise that you can do at home.

Lat Pulldown

Men: helps to develop those big shoulders and that attractive triangle in your upper back. Women: helps you pull your shoulders back to improve your posture and your overall shape.

At a gym, this is done with a long bar, usually suspended from a pulley over your head. Space your arms equally apart on the bar and sit down on a bench. Lean back about 10 degrees and pull the bar straight down to your breast bone, arching your chest up to the bar as it is about to touch your chest.

At home, use the elastic bands that are sold for this purpose; they can be attached to the wall or a doorknob. Read the instructions carefully.

Do three sets of 10 to 15 repetitions each, with only a 30-second rest period in between sets. Men who want to build bulk will need to use gym equipment starting at a weight of between 40 and 70 pounds and building up to 90 to 110 pounds over six weeks. These are general guidelines; you will need to determine the best weight for you.

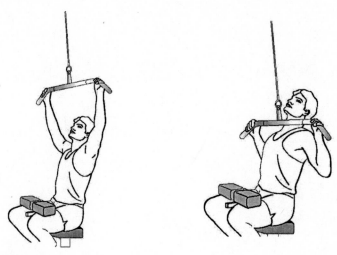

Lat pulldown

Triceps Pushdown

Tones flabby upper arms. While the biceps are important, the triceps fill up that difficult arm area that can flap in the wind if you have too much fat or loose skin there. This muscle group has three heads, as the name implies, and once you master the basic triceps pushdown, you can consult a fitness magazine to learn exercises that work each head of this muscle. For now, here is the basic exercise.

The triceps can be built up by pushing down on a pulley bar in a gym. The straight bar hangs down at a 90 degree angle, and you stand up about a foot away and push the bar down so that when you hold the bar in this position, your elbow is at a 90 degree angle. Let the bar rise slowly up to its original position, then press down in a circular motion, twisting your wrist downward as you push down. Don't push the bar down any further than the 90-degree angle.

To work out at home, choose two dumbbells between 5 and 15 pounds that you can comfortably lift. While lying flat on a mat or a weight bench, hold the dumbbells in each hand with your arms straight up. Lower the

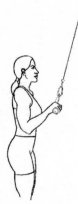

Triceps pushdown at gym

weight slowly, bending at the elbow, until your elbow is at a 90 degree angle and your forearms are nearly parallel to the floor. Now slowly straighten your arm, raising the dumbbells.

Do three sets of 10 to 15 repetitions with only a 30-second rest period in between sets.

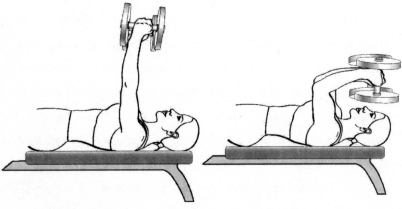

Triceps pushdown at home

Biceps Curl

This exercise builds the most famous of all muscles: the biceps. With more advanced exercises found in fitness magazines, you can build up the two separate heads or parts of this muscle. Women may want to use lighter weights and more repetitions if they want a less muscular look, but

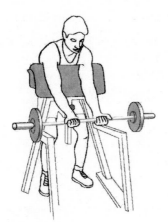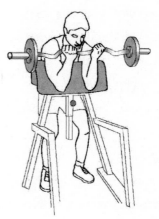

Biceps curl at gym

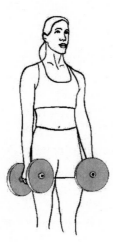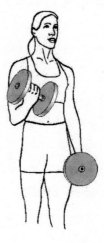

Biceps curl

small biceps on a woman are healthier and more attractive than pencil-thin arms.

This exercise works best if you concentrate on one arm at a time.

Choose dumbbells between 5 and 20 pounds that you can hold easily without straining your wrists. Without bending your wrist, slowly move one weight up until your arm is bent as far as it can go. Then lower the weight slowly and deliberately. You will be stretching your muscle fibers on the way down, causing the mild inflammation or burning needed to build more muscle, and it is especially important to go slowly for the last few repetitions of each set.

Do three sets of 10 to 15 repetitions with each arm, taking only a 30-second rest period in between sets.

Chest Press

The muscles of the chest wall suspend the breast tissue, and in both women and men, a well-developed chest improves overall body shape. There are chest muscles in the mid-, upper, and lower chest, and they can be isolated by doing chest presses at an incline or flat on the bench. The upper and midchest muscles are working when you use an incline of about 45 degrees, and the mid- and lower chest are working when you do your chest presses on a flat bench. Some machines will vary the grip, allowing you to concentrate on different muscle groups.

The basic chest press can be done on a bench press machine or on a weight bench with the arms held apart at about shoulder width. With each repetition, lower the bar to your sternum slowly and raise the weight slowly to get maximum benefit.

Do three sets of 10 to 15 repetitions, with only a 30-second rest period in between sets.

If you don't have access to this equipment, use dumbbells that weigh

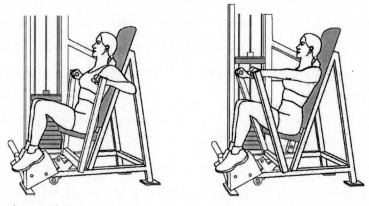

Chest press at gym

between 10 and 30 pounds, as desired. Lie on a flat bench with the dumb-bells in your hands. Start with your elbows at your side and your arms at 90-degree angles and simply push upward, straightening your arm. Return slowly to the starting position.

Repeat three sets of 12 repetitions each. Count to two on the upward movement and to four on the downward movement to make sure you're going slowly enough.

Progressive exercise is a technique that uses heavier weights and

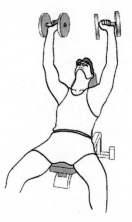

Chest press at home

fewer repetitions to build muscle bulk and then alternates this technique with routines that build power, flexibility, or endurance. Over the first twelve weeks of exercise, you don't need to worry about using progressive exercise techniques, which are described more fully in the Appendix with scientific references. Studies show you will get the same average benefit from just the usual routine of three sets of 8 to 10 repetitions at 60 or 70 percent of your personal one-repetition maximum for that exercise. If at this point you still want to build more muscle, do three sets of 8 to 10 repetitions, increasing the weight each time by 5 pounds per dumbbell until you can only do 6 to 8 repetitions (see the Appendix for more about progressive exercise, which is scientifically the most advanced method to build muscle effectively).

If you just want to tone up and not build muscle, use a weight that is about half as heavy as you could lift comfortably. Do three sets of 15 repetitions.

Chest Fly

This is another great exercise for the chest muscles because it lifts up the pectoral muscles that suspend the breasts in both men and women. You'll improve the shape of your chest and have a more youthful look.

This can be done with dumbbells and a weight bench. Start out with dumbbells in the 10- to 30-pound range for muscle building, and lighter than that if you simply want to tone your chest.

Start out with the bench at a 45-degree incline, and hold the weights straight up. Lower the weights away from the center in a semicircle, stopping at just about the level of your chest. Then bring the weights together again.

Do three sets of 8 to 10 repetitions. This will give you a comfortable burn in your chest muscles as you do the last few repetitions.

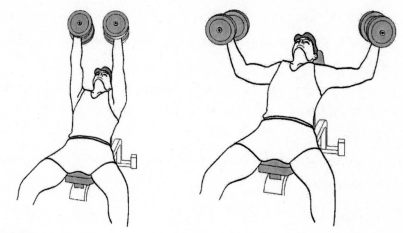

Chest fly

Seated Lateral Raise

This exercise builds a number of muscles around the shoulder, including the deltoid, which in both women and men gives a nicely contoured shape to the shoulder.

This exercise is safest if done while sitting on a bench. If you do it while standing, bend your knees slightly and be careful not to use too

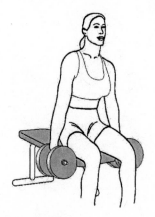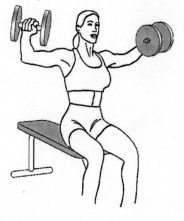

Seated lateral raise

much weight or to jerk the weight upward. Choose dumbbells that are in the 3- to 8-pound range to start and that you can handle very comfortably.

Start with your arms at your sides, keeping your elbows slightly bent. Lift your arms sideways to shoulder height, rotating the weight from your shoulders.

Do three sets of 10 to 15 repetitions, with only a 30-second rest period in between sets.

Reverse Crunch

For great-looking abdominal muscles, you can do stomach crunches or sit-ups. However, for the lower stomach, you need to do special exercises that exercise the abdominal muscles below the belly button. While dieting has a lot to do with getting rid of a pot belly, this exercise can help by toning these muscles.

I wear a weight-lifting belt to protect my back when I do this exercise, and I like to stretch my lower back by rolling backward on the floor before

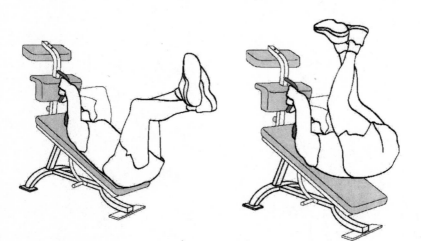

Reverse crunch

starting. If you have a back problem, consult with your doctor or fitness instructor before doing this exercise.

Lie flat on the ground or on a downward incline bench. Extend your legs, then lift them by bending your knees to your chest. Do this quickly, and increase your number of repetitions from 20 to 50 or more with practice.

Leg Raise or Leg Press

If you want nice-looking upper thighs, it is important to work all the muscle groups around the thigh. In addition, these muscles support the knees, so strengthening them helps to protect your knees. Finally, these are large muscles, so increasing their size can really help increase the number of calories you burn every day. If you spend your days sitting in an office or sitting in a car, these muscles are not being used sufficiently, and they are often ignored in weight-lifting exercises because people tend to concentrate on the chest and arms.

At home, do leg raises as follows. If desired, attach two 5-pound ankle weights to one of your legs. You may also want to wear a weight-lifting belt to protect your lower back.

Lie flat on your back and slowly raise your weighted leg 20 times to an angle of about 45 degrees from the floor. Next, lie on your side and raise that leg 20 times to about a 60-degree angle from the floor. Then, lie flat on

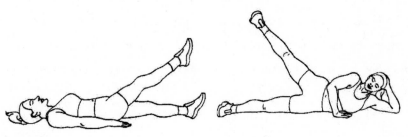

Leg raise

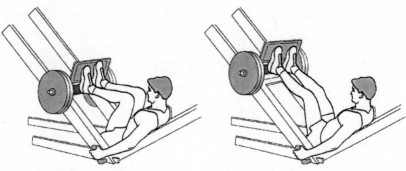

Leg press at gym

your stomach and raise that leg 20 times to about a 30-degree angle from the floor. Switch the weights to the opposite leg and repeat the series.

You can also get good toning of the quadriceps (the large muscle group on the front aspect of the thigh) by doing a greater number of repetitions (between 50 and 100) with no weights.

At a gym, do leg presses on the leg press machine. Most of these machines have you sit in a chair and press a large plate connected to a pulley. Be sure you are using the leg press machine correctly, and pay attention to any pain or discomfort in your knees while doing this exercise. It is a great way to build the quadriceps.

Sit-ups and Abdominal Crunches

You have probably seen the TV commercials in which people build six-packs on their stomachs by using expensive equipment of various kinds. The Federal Trade Commission has determined that all these claims are bogus, and that you can make just as much progress doing sit-ups or abdominal crunches. Of course, there are lots of different opinions about how to do them correctly.

I have found that the most effective sit-ups are those that isolate your abdominal muscles. Lie flat on your back with your hands behind your

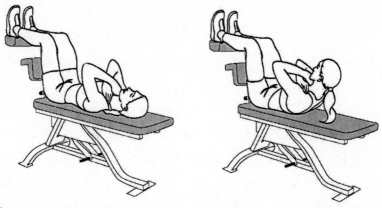

Sit-up

head and your knees bent. Keep your feet flat on the floor, or set them on a chair or bench to increase the difficulty and effectiveness. Slowly raise your head off the floor until you have raised it up as much as possible. Lower your head slowly until you are lying flat again. It is important to go down slowly to obtain maximum muscle-building benefit. Do 20 repetitions at first, and increase to 100 or more.

Crunches are done from the same position; just don't lower your head all the way to the floor on the downward motion. Go about two-thirds of the way, and then go back up again.

There is an ongoing discussion about whether crunches or sit-ups are better. It is a matter of personal preference, and I suggest you find an exercise that you prefer so that you will do it every day. Sit-ups and crunches can be varied with advanced techniques such as bending, holding a weight plate on your chest, or doing them on a reverse-inclined bench. For now, just get started with a simple and personal choice. For most people, the crunch gives them permission to do a more restricted exercise that is more comfortable than a full sit-up.

Calf Raise

Good calf muscles are important for keeping your body supported if you stand a lot, especially in high heels. They support the knees from below and help with lifting and climbing stairs.

At the gym, use a machine with pads that fit on your shoulders while you stand on a platform a few inches off the ground. Rise up on your toes, then slowly drop back down. The shoulder pads cushion your shoulders and upper back as you push up between 20 and 50 pounds with your calves. Since your toes are on the machine while your ankles are free to move, you do the movement more easily than if you're standing flat on the ground.

If you don't have a gym, simply stand near a wall for support and do the same movement, rising up on your toes and then going back down to the floor. You may be able to do more repetitions with no weights, but try holding light dumbbells to progress the exercise and build some shapely calves.

Do three sets of 10 to 15 repetitions, with only a 30-second rest period in between sets.

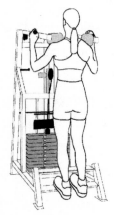 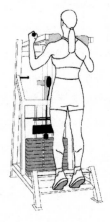

Calf raise

Planning What to Eat Before and After Exercise

It is hard to perform exercises when you are still digesting food, and it is equally hard to exercise if you skipped your last meal. So, it is important to be careful about what you eat both before and after exercise.

If you eat too much, your intestines will steal blood flow from your muscles and you may end up getting a cramp. You should not exercise for about 30 minutes after a meal, and you should avoid a heavy protein meal just before exercising.

The best thing to eat before exercise is a light meal of easy-to-digest carbohydrates (fruits and vegetables) and a small amount of protein. A great choice is a protein shake made with berries that contain lots of antioxidants, such as blueberries. I usually exercise in the morning 30 minutes after having my soy shake with fruit and a cup of coffee.

Loading up with carbohydrates is not necessary if you have been eating normally for the past few days. You are not trying to win a gold medal in the marathon; you just want enough energy for your exercise session. A carbohydrate snack before you start will give you some energy to get going, especially if you're working out in the late afternoon.

When you are done exercising, it is very important that you eat a snack such as a protein bar or protein drink with both protein and carbohydrates providing 100 to 200 calories within 30 minutes, and that you drink enough water to restore your fluid balance. The carbs will restore muscle glycogen, the protein will provide amino acids to help build muscle tissue, and the water will help you maintain normal circulation to the muscles.

Thirst is an excellent monitor of how much fluid you need. Drinking water works just fine for hydration, although you may prefer a special sports drink if you've been sweating profusely during your workout. To check how much water you need, weigh yourself both before and after your workout. For each pound of weight you lose, drink two 8-ounce glasses of water. If you don't feel like weighing yourself and you are having a typical 30-minute workout, just get in the habit of drinking two glasses of water or finish a 16-ounce water bottle while you exercise to stay hydrated.

If you don't feel like eating solid carbohydrates and protein foods after you exercise, a shake or protein bar is a great way to get easy nutrition into your system. Some companies sell muscle-recovery bars or even gels designed for this purpose. The protein acts to minimize the pain and burning in your muscles and joints by reducing the breakdown of muscle protein after you exercise. Certain amino acids called "branched chain amino acids" can have a specially beneficial effect on maintaining muscle protein stores during exercise, and these bars are rich in these particular amino acids.

Eating colorful fruits and vegetables provides phytonutrients and antioxidants that help protect your muscle cells from excessive oxidation as you exercise. As I've mentioned, some mild inflammation is helpful in building muscle. However, part of the purpose of the rest period is to repair this good damage and build muscle. The good part of the damage is not affected by nutrition, but eating a lot of antioxidant-rich foods can help keep your muscles from getting sore from excessive damage between workouts. In addition to eating fruits and vegetables, some antioxidant supplements, including vitamin E, have been shown to reduce excess damage to muscle fibers following exercise.

Putting Your Exercise Program Together

You may burn a lot of calories in the gym, but you can lose even more weight through the freedom from cravings that you get when you're addicted to exercise. In fact, the blood levels of the pleasure hormone endorphin have been shown to increase just prior to exercise. After you've followed an exercise program for a couple of weeks, you may notice that you feel out of sorts when for some reason you don't have time to exercise. This is the withdrawal reaction from the healthy exercise addiction.

Perform your cardiovascular exercise after your weight-training workout or on alternate days so you have plenty of strength to finish your cardio routine. Start with a 5-minute warm-up, then stretch, follow with weight training, and your aerobic workout. The bottom line: Do some sort of aerobic exercise every day—your body will thank you.

The rest periods are taken for each muscle group. So you can exercise every day by rotating the muscle groups that are being exercised. In my case, I rotate so that I do chest and triceps, then back and biceps, and finally legs and shoulders. Each day I do aerobics and I try to exercise six of seven days.

When I travel I try to maintain my routine as best I can. The equipment I mentioned earlier can be found in many hotels, so when you are on a business trip just pack a pair of lightweight track shoes, a pair of socks, some gym shorts, and a T-shirt. If your hotel doesn't have a gym, you can find one in the neighborhood and pay a guest fee.

However, remember that exercise is meant to be fun and an addictive behavior—not a chore.

L.A. Shape Enhancers

Supplements and Herbal Approaches

At this point, you have implemented the six simple steps to success that I promised you at the beginning. Step 7 provides you with some advanced nutrition information and some special strategies you can use to maximize your success when you hit roadblocks along the way to your personal best shape.

You can maximize your health by adding supplements to a healthy diet. I will evaluate the evidence and suggest proper doses for the vitamin, mineral, and other supplements everyone should consider. I will also tell you about a new class of supplements that extract the phytochemicals from fruits and vegetables and provide these as tablets or in capsules. While some supplements have claimed to jam the whole produce section into a single pill, the supplements I recommend are different and contain about the amount of phytochemicals you would ingest in a single serving of a specific fruit or vegetable featured in the seven colors of health.

When you hit roadblocks along the way, such as reduced energy, too much snacking, or troubling cellulite, you may consider adding an herbal supplement that can help you with these problems. I evaluate the evidence on the safety and effectiveness of the available supplement and herbal approaches to weight loss so you can judge for yourself. However, remember that there are no magic pills that will do the first six steps for you. The supplements in this chapter are called "enhancers" because they may help you change your shape when used together with the rest of your program.

Vitamins and Minerals

For the past fifty years the accepted medical wisdom (and what I was taught in medical school thirty years ago) was that you could get everything you needed for healthy nutrition from the four basic food groups—dairy, grains, fruits and vegetables, and meats, beans, nuts, and cheese. While it is theoretically possible to do this with a well-designed diet, in practice this is rather difficult. Many of us—even if we think we have a good diet—consume inadequate amounts of vitamin C, vitamin E, folic acid, zinc, magnesium, vitamin A, and calcium. Poor intakes of these nutrients have been confirmed by government surveys on the U.S. population. Data from these surveys (known as NHANES III and CSFII) have been used by government advisory groups to establish the dietary recommendations for all Americans.

In fact, there is even more compelling science and bitter experience that has taught us that there are some supplements you really need in order to be healthy, because Americans simply don't consume enough through food sources. A serious birth defect called "spina bifida," in which the spinal cords of newborn infants are not fused properly, has been shown to be due to deficiencies of folic acid in pregnant women. Calcium deficiency has been shown to lead to osteoporosis, or thinning of the bones. It's not that you can't find folic acid and calcium in widely available foods, such as dark leafy greens and dairy, but rather that Americans simply don't eat enough of them.

Consumers have been way ahead of the medical profession on this one, and have been taking supplements for at least the past twenty years. In fact, vitamins and mineral supplements are the most common nonprescription pills taken in this country, with about 40 percent of all Americans reporting that they take vitamins.

Vitamins are not a substitute for a healthy diet, but they will help you achieve better overall nutritional health when combined with the typical "good" diet. In fact, studies show that people who remember to take their vitamins in the morning also remember to eat right and go to the gym; the mere act of taking a multivitamin reminds you about your healthy lifestyle. Since it's very hard to eat perfectly every day, especially if you travel, vitamins and minerals will help you consistently get the substances you need for good health.

You have probably read about possible side effects, including toxicity. But these kinds of problems occur only when vitamins are taken far in excess of the recommended dietary allowance, or RDA. For example, with water-soluble vitamins such as the B vitamins, side effects of numbness and tingling on the tongue occur when one B vitamin, such as B_6, is taken at a dose of 500 milligrams, which is a hundred times its RDA. An exception to this rule is vitamin A, which our bodies can make from beta-carotene (which also supplies the orange color in carrots). Studies from the Harvard School of Public Health have shown that taking in excess of 8,500 International Units (IU) a day is associated with osteoporosis. As a result of this study, multivitamin manufacturers have now replaced all or a large portion of their vitamin A with beta-carotene, and some reduce the total amount of vitamin A and beta-carotene to 3,500 IU for safety. You can get all the vitamin A you need from eating vegetables that provide vitamin A from beta-carotene, and the advantage is that your body will only make as much vitamin A as you need.

Say that you consume your recommended daily allowance in vitamins and also eat a healthy diet. What is the downside? You will only take in twice or less the recommended level of any vitamin or mineral, and your body can handle this easily. For each of the vitamins and minerals recommended, there is a biological rationale and a safety factor that is more than generous. Not only are vitamins safe, but they promote your good health.

Start with a simple program of vitamin and mineral supplementation and build up. If you go overboard and try to take too many pills, there is a chance you will burn out and stop taking the important ones. The following list gives vitamins, minerals, and herbal dietary supplements in their order of importance, given the strength of the medical and scientific evidence for taking them.

In general, the level of scientific evidence for vitamins and minerals is stronger than for herbs, simply because the former have been studied much more thoroughly. The growing acceptance of vitamin and mineral supplements by the medical profession is evidenced by recent articles in both the *Journal of the American Medical Association* and the *New England Journal of Medicine* recommending a daily multivitamin supplement. It is important to know the quality of the products you are purchasing, since the FDA does not take responsibility for either the science behind supplements or their manufacturing at this time. Most vitamins are produced according to well-established standards similar to those used for over-the-counter drugs such as aspirin. The FDA recently issued some guidelines for good manufacturing practices that should improve the quality of herbal supplements in the future. At UCLA my colleagues and I use sophisticated methods to examine the chemical profile of herbs, and in many cases we grow the plants we are studying in a greenhouse. We then measure the actual contents of active compounds in our herbal extracts before studying them so that our results are standardized. As manufacturing practices improve over the next few years, more producers of dietary supplements should be using these types of methods. You should check the particular supplements you are taking to see what methods are being used by the manufacturer to guarantee quality. This information should be available on their website or by calling the manufacturer.

The Core Group of Vitamins and Minerals

Here are my basic four vitamin supplements to complement the so-called basic four food groups. Remember, you're basing your diet on food plus pills, not food versus pills. Foods provide lots of fiber, and families of compounds called "phytochemicals" in fruits, vegetables, and grains. Some newer supplements are providing concentrated extracts of these phytochemicals not available in traditional multivitamins. However, you should also eat a healthy diet of colorful fruits and vegetables, since vitamins are no excuse for eating a lousy diet.

Here are the recommended daily allowances for some of the most important vitamins and minerals. I recommend that you take a *multivitamin/multimineral* every day that conforms to this list:

Natural carotenoids from an algae source, such as D. Salina	5000 IU per day
Lutein from marigolds	250 mcg
Lycopene from tomato	300 mcg
Vitamin C	60 mg
Vitamin D	400 IU

Vitamin E (alpha tocopherol)	30 IU
Thiamin	1.5 mg
Riboflavin	1.7 mg
Niacin	20 mg
Vitamin B6	2 mg
Vitamin B12	6 mcg
Biotin	100 mcg
Pantothenic acid	10 mg
Calcium	167 mg
Iron	10 mg
Iodine	150 mcg
Magnesium	100 mg
Zinc	15 mg
Copper	2 mg
Selenium	20 mcg
Manganese	2 mg
Chromium	120 mcg
Potassium	80 mg
Vanadium	10 mcg
Tin	10 mcg
Silicon	2 mg

This is the ideal content of a general multivitamin; for more optimized vitamin supplementation, see Step 7.

Beyond the daily multivitamin/multimineral, there is evidence that individual vitamins and minerals may have health benefits. Here are some suggestions for additional individual vitamin supplementation:

VITAMIN E

400 IU per day. A standard multivitamin/multimineral contains only about the RDA of 15 to 30 IU of vitamin E. This is just enough to avoid a deficiency, but it is not enough for you to gain vitamin E's antioxidant benefits. Between 200 and 800 IU have been shown to have the greatest benefit for immune function for the elderly and heart disease prevention.

VITAMIN C

500 mg per day. You can prevent scurvy with only 20 mg per day, but the RDA was increased to 60 mg per day in part to recognize the benefits of vitamin C as an antioxidant. If you eat enough fruits and vegetables, you will get a good amount of vitamin C. Just a handful of strawberries or an orange will fulfill your RDA. The body is able to store about 1,500 mg in all, and you lose about 45 mg per day in your urine.

Vitamin C is rapidly cleared from the body by the liver and is excreted in the urine. At doses above 250 mg per day you start to find oxalate (a breakdown product of vitamin C) in the urine. The most common doses taken by individuals range between 250 mg and 1,000 mg per day of vitamin C in addition to what you get from fruits and vegetables. At doses over 1,500 mg per day, some people will get kidney stones made from the oxalate excreted into the urine. I generally recommend that if you choose to take a separate vitamin C supplement that you limit yourself to 500 mg per day.

CALCIUM

1,000 to 1,500 mg per day. Ancient man consumed about 1,600 mg per day in plant foods, and so we evolved to absorb only a fraction of our dietary calcium. As we age, we have a decreased ability to absorb calcium because

The L.A. Shape Diet

of decreased acid section by the stomach lining. Taking calcium with a meal in the form of calcium carbonate will work well, but you may want to take calcium citrate, since this form does not require stomach acid, and is more efficiently absorbed than calcium carbonate (50 percent versus 30 percent).

SELENIUM

50 to 200 mcgs per day in the form of selenomethionine. Selenium is an essential mineral necessary for the functioning of an enzyme called "glutathione peroxidase," which protects our DNA from oxidant damage. In one study, patients received supplements of selenium at 200 mcgs per day, and researchers observed a reduced rate of prostate and breast cancer. Since the study was designed to test the effects of selenium on skin cancer, additional studies are now being done to confirm these results.

GREEN TEA EXTRACT CAPSULES

250 mg to 500 mg, containing about 100 to 160 mg of EGCG (epigallocatechingallate). Green tea contains chemicals called "polyphenols" that are very strong antioxidants (and EGCG is thought to be one of the most active polyphenols). In some experiments, where the ability to protect DNA from oxidation was studied, green tea was 2,500 times as potent an antioxidant as beta-carotene.

The polyphenols appear to be able to enhance nervous system activity at the level of the fat cell, causing it to release more fat. Since caffeine occurs naturally in green tea extract, it has been difficult to separate the effects of green tea from caffeine in humans. However, a recent study by Abdul Dulloo and his group gave subjects green tea extract capsules three times per day. These capsules contained green tea, which naturally had 150 mg caffeine, and 375 mg of catechin polyphenols. Subjects spent three 24-hour periods in an energy chamber, during which they received the above mentioned green tea extract, 150 mg of caffeine alone, or a placebo. The amount of energy burned per day by the subjects was higher by 4.5 percent in those who received green tea compared to a placebo, and 3.2 percent higher than when the same dose of caffeine was given alone. In addition, fat burning was increased. The net effect attributable to green tea could be estimated at approximately 80 calories per day.

Green tea extract capsules that concentrate the polyphenols from 4 to 6 cups of green tea in a single capsule, with reduced caffeine content, are a convenient alternative to drinking 4 to 6 cups of green tea daily. Ongoing research is revealing other potential benefits of green tea. In some studies, green tea keeps tumor cells from growing new blood vessels. Many drug companies are developing expensive agents, called "angiogenesis inhibitors," for this purpose; if given to a cancer patient, they have to be taken for life. A natural, less expensive product such as green tea would obviously be more desirable for the public than an expensive drug, if it could be proven to have the same benefits.

While both green tea and black tea are naturally caffeinated and both can be decaffeinated, there are some differences in the polyphenols found in green tea and black tea. Green tea is made by heating or steaming tea leaves just after they are picked. If green tea leaves are allowed to dry without heating or steaming, they turn brown, and the catechins they contain are then chemically linked in the drying tea leaves to form larger chemicals called "theaflavins." The steaming of the leaves inactivates the normal protein in the cells of the tea leaves, which acts to break down tea catechins as they are dried. Given the nature of green tea, it is not surprising that the levels of catechins vary greatly among different brands of green tea and black tea. The time and temperature at which you brew your tea will also affect the levels of catechins. So I recommend drinking green or black tea if you enjoy it, but that you take a capsule to get the health benefits of the tea.

ALPHA LIPOIC ACID

20 to 50 mg a day. This antioxidant, in combination with N-acetylcarnitine (another antioxidant), has been shown to slow the aging of laboratory mice in research conducted at the University of California at Berkeley. Because it is found only in minute amounts in foods, taking supplemental alpha lipoic acid makes sense. In diabetics, 300 to 600 mg a day has been found to be beneficial for treating the nerve damage often associated with diabetes.

UBIQUINONE (COENZYME Q_{10})

30 mg per day. This enzyme seems to have a special role in muscle cells, including those within the heart. It concentrates in the particles carrying LDL cholesterol in the blood and protects the cholesterol from oxidation. This action helps prevent the inflammation in the blood vessel walls that promotes atherosclerosis.

PYCNOGENOL

100 mg per day. This is an extract of the bark of the French pine tree. The main components are phenolic compounds, including catechins similar to those found in green tea, and condensed flavonoids, including anthocyanidins and proanthocyanidins. These anti-inflammatory agents act as strong antioxidants and reduce the tendency toward excessive blood clotting that occurs in many overweight individuals.

PHYTOCHEMICAL SUPPLEMENTS

A number of supplements have tried to incorporate the health values that are being discovered for phytochemicals from fruits and vegetables.

The first of these supplements claimed to provide chemicals from a number of dried vegetables. They were not at all credible, as they claimed to compress the whole produce section into a single capsule or pill. When you try to combine all of the most common phytochemicals into a single tablet, you cannot get the amounts of these phytochemicals needed to impact your health.

Some well-known multivitamin capsules add small amounts of phytochemicals such as lycopene or lutein. While it is great that they have the ability to increase public awareness of these phytochemicals, the amounts of these phytochemicals cannot substitute for single servings of the corresponding vegetables.

It is possible to concentrate tomato oil into a capsule so that the mixture of phytochemicals found in a tomato can be supplemented in a capsule. By combining this capsule with others containing the major phytochemicals found in each of the seven color groups, it is possible to assemble a phytonutrient pack of seven tablets—one for each color group that could deliver the amounts of phytochemicals approximating those found in one serving of each of the seven colors of health. This type of convenience pack of seven tablets would provide a valuable supplement if you are not sure you can get your seven servings every day. In addition, studies have shown that the levels of active compounds in fruits and vegetables vary depending on where and how they are grown and harvested. Studies have demonstrated wide store-to-store and region-to-region variations in the content of isothiocyanate in broccoli samples from grocery store produce sections. These types of supplements will also lead to new research on the health benefits of fruits and vegetables and may well be the new vitamins of the twenty-first century.

Dietary Supplements and Herbs for Weight Loss

Some herbal products for weight reduction and maintenance may be helpful only when combined with healthy diet and lifestyle changes. The safety and efficacy of some available herbal products for weight reduction remain major issues. In 2003 the FDA finally issued provisional good manufacturing practices—more than ten years after passage of the legislation that mandated this action. Responsible manufacturers are moving to come into compliance with these guidelines.

Given these considerations, it is vital that patients who plan to use supplements choose products from reliable manufacturers, read labels carefully, follow instructions on proper dosage, and learn which products are efficacious. The advice and supervision of an informed primary care physician can certainly minimize the risk of adverse side effects and maximize the chances for benefit. In order to monitor safety retroactively, the FDA relies on the reporting of adverse effects by physicians as part of a program called MEDWATCH, which was originally designed for postmarketing surveillance of prescription drugs. Unfortunately, this method has significant drawbacks because it's difficult to confirm a causal relationship between the use of a particular botanical dietary supplement and a reported side effect, especially when the side effect is a disease such as heart disease that is more common in obese individuals, regardless of whether or not they are taking a dietary supplement.

CAFFEINE

You may not think of your morning cup of coffee as an herb for weight loss, but caffeine can increase pulse rate and metabolism. Many of us have a cup of coffee in the morning along with our high-protein breakfast, and there is nothing wrong with that. However, I am currently reviewing the use of caffeine in dietary supplements as pills or teas that can be used beyond the simple morning cup of coffee.

Caffeine in an oral dose of 250 mg increased the release of fat from fat cells as measured by the levels of free fatty acids in the blood of both obese and lean humans, compared to a water placebo. Oxygen consumption is increased in normal subjects who are given caffeine orally, compared to glucose as a control. Oxygen consumption, which is a measure of total calories burned, and fat breakdown were also increased after about 280 mg of caffeine from coffee compared to a decaffeinated control, both after fasting and after a mixed meal.

Caffeine causes increased heat production, which is released through an increase in skin temperature—a reaction that is familiar to anyone who has consumed several cups of coffee at one sitting. When different individuals are given a dose of 150 mg of caffeine, the observed increase in their calorie burning will vary. The amount that it increases can be used to predict how much weight each individual will lose on a diet and exercise program. So caffeine can be used to identify those individuals with "good metabolism." Also, increased doses of caffeine cause proportionally increased amounts of calorie burning in the same individual. In short, there is scientific evidence that supports the use of caffeine in weight reduction.

Several studies have addressed the safety of caffeine. The positive association between heavy coffee drinking and elevated cholesterol found in some studies is explained by factors other than the caffeine found in coffee, since caffeine consumption in the form of tea or cola has no effect on cholesterol. A clinical trial with 288 healthy subjects evaluated the effects on blood pressure of a single 200 mg-per-day dose of caffeine, compared to a placebo. Blood pressure is measured as two numbers (e.g., 120/80). The first number is the systolic pressure (the highest average pressure to which your arteries are exposed by the pumping of the heart), and the second number is the diastolic pressure (the low tide after the heart relaxes), measured as pressures in millimeters of mercury (abbreviated mm Hg). Caffeine gave a 2.2-mm-Hg rise in diastolic blood pressure, which was felt to be clinically insignificant. There was no change in pulse rate or systolic blood pressure. Similarly, the negative effects of drinking more than two cups of coffee per day on bone loss in women is associated with factors other than the caffeine in coffee. So I would recommend no more than two cups of coffee per day whether or not it is decaffeinated, and that you take caffeine in the form of supplements or teas to which caffeine has been added as a weight-loss aid. The FDA approves caffeine for sale without a prescription for use as a stimulant by people twelve years of age or older at a dose up to 200 mg every 3 hours (1,600 mg/d) and as an ingredient in pain medications, which gives further support to its safety.

CAPSAICIN FROM CHILI PEPPERS

Capsaicin from chili peppers and red bell peppers has been shown to stimulate fat breakdown and the generation of heat. If you have ever eaten a superhot habañero pepper, this will come as no surprise to you. The hotness of compounds in chili peppers is rated (as is a heater in your home) by heat-producing units called Scoville Units or S.U. People have varying reactions to the same S.U. level; it depends on how often they have eaten chili peppers in the past. If they are used to chili peppers, their bodies release endorphin, the pleasure hormone, upon eating them. The exact mechanism for this effect is not known. There are also reports of modest weight loss in subjects who consume chili peppers regularly. So, if you have a supplement containing chili peppers, you should use it to help you lose additional weight when and if you hit a rough spot in your efforts to do so. You can also add these spices to your healthy foods and get some of the same benefits.

CONJUGATED LINOLEIC ACID

Conjugated linoleic acid, or CLA, is a fatty acid that has been shown to lower cholesterol and inhibit heart disease and cancer in animals. It is found in trace amounts in cheese and milk, and when cows are given extra vegetable oils, the amount of CLA in their milk increases. CLA can also be made by a simple chemical reaction in the laboratory. Synthetic CLA is a mixture of two different chemical forms of this compound; one, the so-called 9–11 form, is thought to be responsible for the anticancer activity in the animal studies discussed earlier, and the other, the 10–12 form, is thought to be responsible for the loss of body fat. If all this chemistry makes little sense to you—don't worry. You just need to know that CLA is a compound that is still under study for its effects on cancer and heart disease.

In studies designed to explore the effects of CLA on weight loss, mice fed a diet supplemented with 0.5 percent by weight of CLA at constant calories develop 60 percent less body fat than animals fed a control diet. This decrease in body fat is most likely due to a combination of reduced fat deposition, increased release of fat from fat cells, and increased fat breakdown by the body. However, studies in humans to treat obesity suggest that CLA may not work in humans. Further research is necessary to demonstrate the safety and effects of this supplement. At this time, I would not recommend CLA for weight loss, given the evidence.

GARCINIA CAMBOGIA (HYDROXYCITRIC ACID)

Garcinia cambogia is a small, sweet, purple fruit, commonly known as Malabar tamarind. The fruit rind contains hydroxycitric acid (HCA), similar to the citric acid found in citrus fruit. Dried, thin pieces of the rind are added to curries or substituted for lime in the cuisines of India, Laos, Malaysia, and Burma to make the foods seem more filling.

Hydroxycitric acid works by inhibiting lipogenesis—the process by which the body converts carbohydrates into fat—by temporarily inhibiting ATP:citrate lyase, the enzyme that converts excess glucose to fat.

A recent study published in the *International Journal of Obesity* measured decreased snacking by giving twenty-four healthy and overweight subjects either about 8 ounces of tomato juice or about 8 ounces of tomato juice with 300 mg of HCA, 1 hour before lunch and dinner and once at 2 hours after dinner, three times daily, for six weeks. After two weeks, results showed 24-hour calorie intake was reduced significantly (15 to 30 percent) compared to a placebo, with sustained satiety, mainly because of a significant decrease (about 41 percent) in between-meal snacking. Taking a supplement of garcinia cambogia of the right form is something I would recommend to defend against too much snacking.

Fighting Cellulite

Women trying to reduce cellulite have a cosmetic goal in mind and may or may not care about actual fat and weight loss. The cause of the dimpling seen with cellulite is an increased growth of fibrous boundaries in the fat tissue under the skin in the rear thigh. Cellulite usually develops with the weight gain of pregnancy at any age, but it can occur in women with lower-body fat who are in their early twenties.

The cosmetic goal of reducing and smoothing thigh fat can be approached with either a topical cream or with liposuction. In all cases, women should try to use topical creams before even considering surgery. Surgery is a last resort and must be done at a time when diet and exercise habits are under excellent control, or you risk undoing your expensive surgery by gaining back your fat through poor diet.

Local application to the fat cells of substances that stimulate the release of fat from fat cells has the potential to reduce the size of the treated fat cells. The potential of benefit of this scientific knowledge was demonstrated in a study of women where different agents that release fat from fat cells in the laboratory were tested. Using one thigh as a control, isoproterenol injections (a beta receptor stimulator), forskolin ointment (a direct stimulator of adenylate cyclase), yohimbine ointment (an alpha-2 receptor inhibitor), and aminophylline (an inhibitor of phosphodiesterase and the adenosine receptor) showed more girth loss from the treated thigh than the control. Treatments were given once daily, five days a week, for one month. These results of injections led to other studies examining the use of creams, which is a more practical approach to losing cellulite. In a six-week study with 10 percent aminophylline ointment in twenty-three subjects, a five-week study with 2 percent aminophylline cream in eleven subjects, and a five-week study with 0.5 percent aminophylline cream in twelve subjects, none of the creams were more effective than the 0.5 percent aminophylline, which showed more than a 3-cm difference between the treated and untreated thighs. However, a twelve-week study using a similar design was unable to reproduce these results for aminophylline cream.

An oral product containing gingko biloba, sweet clover, seaweed, grape seed oil, lecithins, and evening primrose oil has been marketed for the treatment of cellulite. In a two-month placebo-controlled trial, this product offered no reduction in body weight, fat content, thigh circumference, hip circumference, or dimply appearance of the fat.

Because of the great interest in these creams, some ineffective products have been marketed and in one famous case, removed from the market by the government because the cream was found to be ineffective. This is an area of ongoing research and these creams should be considered as cosmetic approaches that remove a small amount of fat. The best advice is to do as much as you can with Steps 1 through 6, including accepting your body shape once you have done all you can to enhance your shape.

SUMMARY OF EFFICACY AND SAFETY OF WEIGHT-LOSS APPROACHES

Weight-Loss Approach	Does It Work?	Evidence of Safety?
Caffeine	Good—clinical trial	Good
Green tea catechins	Good—metabolic study	Excellent
Capsaicin	Good—clinical trial	Excellent
Conjugated linoleic acid	Weak—clinical trial	Questionable
Garcinia cambogia	Poor—clinical trial	Excellent
Chromium picolinate	Ineffective	Good
Betahydroxymethylbutyrate	Ineffective for weight loss	Good
Topical fat reduction	Cosmetic only	Excellent

It is your right to choose to take the supplements in the list shown as long as they are not taken off the market by the FDA for safety concerns, as was the case with phenylpropanolamine, which was the active ingredient in the original Dexatrim, Accutrim, and similar over-the-counter slimming products. Your right to choose a supplement is guaranteed by law in a bill called the Dietary Supplement Health Education Act, which was passed by the U.S. Congress in 1994. There are those in Congress who want to change the law or eliminate it altogether, which would be a tragedy in my view. It would throw out the baby with the bathwater, and eliminate our chances of doing the science that is needed to develop the full public health potential of herbal dietary supplements.

I suggest that you become as informed a consumer as possible. The National Center for Complementary and Alternative Medicine has a website (www.nccam.org), as does the UCLA Center for Human Nutrition (uclanutrition.org). Try these sites for more information and the latest breakthroughs in research on herbal dietary supplements.

Principles of Dieting and Your Body Shape

In this chapter, I discuss the unchanging laws that determine how your body controls its shape and body fat. Nature has put very real systems into place to keep us from starving, and I don't know of any animal that has evolved to eat whatever it wants and still be able to lose weight. Our genes are programmed to deal with things we have to face every day. Many of our genes are occupied in fighting off the damaging effects of the oxygen we breathe. These antioxidant defenses are an important part of our fight against disease. Being overweight with an apple shape puts extra stress on this defense system, because fat cells make hormones called "cytokines" that stimulate inflammation and the production of oxygen free radicals in your body. So when you overeat and gain weight, you are doing something nature was not prepared to accommodate.

We all have friends who seem to be able to eat whatever they want and not gain weight. This is an illusion. They may not gain weight as easily as you do, but they will eventually gain weight if they eat too much and exercise too little. A study done a number of years ago with prisoners in Vermont showed that lean prisoners did not gain exactly the amount you would expect when overfed. For every extra 3,500 calories per week they ate, they should have gained 1 pound. In fact, what was seen was that they gained only about 60 percent of the weight they were expected to gain.

This ability to burn off some calories when you are overfed was discovered in the early 1900s by German scientists, who called it *Luxuskonsumption*. Although this looks like something that ought to be stamped on the trunk of a German sports car, its existence has been confirmed by many other scientists around the world. Unfortunately, it is a relatively weak mechanism when faced with the sea of high-fat and high-sugar foods, combined with the physical inactivity that's so common in our culture.

In this book, I have asked you to do some unnatural things. I have asked you to eat in a healthy way and to exercise. This is not a great sales pitch when compared to the many claims you hear every day about the magical ways to lose weight. If any of these were true, I would have included them in my book. Having been at this for more than twenty-five years, I can assure you that there is nothing out there that can deliver on some of the outrageous promises you hear.

So, here it is: Dieting works according to certain principles that are built into the laws of nature. If you know this stuff, please feel free to skim over it. On the other hand, if you have been watching a lot of cable television paid programming (otherwise known as "infomercials"), you have been promised that these principles don't count. You have been told you can eat whatever you want and still lose weight. You have been promised supplements that will help you lose weight while you sleep, no matter what diet you are following. You have been promised exercises that don't take effort. All you have to do is sit back in your pajamas and attach a device to your body, and you'll get a six-pack stomach and thin, shapely thighs. There's just one thing you have to do first: call an 800 number and lose weight in the only place that counts to these people—your wallet or purse! Well, here's a quick review of what's really happening in your body and mind.

Principle 1: Energy In = Energy Out + Energy Stored

If you take in fewer calories than your body needs, it will burn some of the its stored protein, fat, and carbohydrate in order to get the energy it needs. When your body gets about 500 fewer calories per day than it needs, either as a result of your eating less or burning more, you will lose 1 pound of weight per week. There are small but significant differences in how efficiently your body can burn or deposit fat, carbohydrate, and protein. These small differences may be why increasing protein intake as a percentage of total calories may help prevent weight regain after weight is lost.

However, in determining your projected rate of weight loss on a diet, it is simply a matter of calories in versus calories out. Eat fewer calories than you burn, and you lose weight. Eat more than you need, and you gain weight. Meal replacements such as the Empowering Shake work by letting you know exactly how many calories you have eaten. This helps you organize your eating, so you have a better idea of how many calories you are consuming each day.

Principle 2: All Diets Are Not Created Equal

Diets vary widely, from those suggesting you could lose weight effectively by simply eating twenty-five fewer pieces of chocolate or walking 2,000 more steps per day to those in which all sugar and carbohydrates or all fats are restricted. However, in order to be safe, a diet must provide the protein you need. If you starve or consume too little protein, your body will take protein from your vital organs and tissues, including your heart muscle. On one of the drastic starvation diets of the 1970s, about eighty women lost so much heart muscle protein that they suffered complications that included abnormal heart rhythms, heart attacks, and death. Without some education, it is easily possible to lose weight in an unhealthy way.

However, some people will try to scare you into thinking that a high-protein diet is unsafe. This is also not true. In the 1980s, a theory called the "Brenner Hypothesis" stated that high-protein intake would lead to kidney failure. This theory was never proven, and plant proteins such as soy protein don't have any deleterious effects on kidney function. Animal proteins can theoretically have some negative effects on kidney function. However, most authorities believe that protein of all types is safe at usual intakes up to about 2 grams per pound of lean body mass. The *L.A. Shape Diet* recommends 1 gram per pound of lean body mass, well within the safe range. When the Zone recommended a diet that contained 30 percent protein (about 1 gram per pound of lean body mass), it was attacked as being too high in protein by the American Dietetic Association, which promoted a diet with 15 percent protein. When I was in medical school thirty years ago, cereals and grains were considered the main dietary staple, so 15 percent was the recommended amount of protein (see the Appendix, the Science of Cereals and Shakes, and elsewhere in this chapter).

The popularity of the Zone led to a resurgence in protein-focused diets, and ultimately the new Atkins high-protein/high-fat indulgence diet.

The history of diet books since the 1970s is one of people looking for some magic trick that will help them lose weight while making only small changes in their usual diet. Let's take a look at some of these diets over the years. In 1972, the first version of the Atkins diet identified carbohydrates as the main problem and proposed a high-protein and high-fat diet. In 1980, the Beverly Hills diet was based on a high intake of expensive fruits and vegetables within a low-fat diet. In 1989, after the Surgeon General's Report featured an almost total concentration on limiting fat in the diet as the cause of both obesity and high fat in the diet, *The Pritikin Weight Loss Breakthrough Diet* was published, and the very-low fat diet was securely in place as the healthy approach.

In 1995, the Zone endorsed eating 30 percent protein and 30 percent fat, compared to the 10 to 15 percent fat recommended by Pritikin and other low-fat gurus. This made food taste better. *Protein Power, Sugar Busters* and the return of the Atkins diet followed, with high fat and high protein. *Eat Right for Your Type* was based on the false premise that blood types determine the best diet for you personally. *The South Beach Diet* basically takes the position that it is not low carbohydrate or low fat, but says that good fats and good carbohydrates are fine. Bread, pasta, potatoes, baked goods, and fruits are restricted for fourteen days, but you are told you can add these back in once you lose weight. Once again, the message is that you can get there simply. "Dr. Phil" takes a different view. His diet is the old-fashioned balanced diet recommended by the USDA decades ago combined with a heavy dose of psychology, which is what he knows best.

None of these diets will hurt you if you stay on them for a few days or weeks, but they waste the opportunity to lose weight successfully and permanently that you get with the L.A. Shape Diet. What's more, constant "on and off" dieting preoccupies a high percentage of the population and uses up a lot of time, energy, and money without producing much happiness. Why do all these diets work for a while and then fail?

Principle 3: You Are Well Adapted to Starvation

It is natural for your body to fight to maintain your weight when you take in fewer calories than you need. Starvation and near-starvation have always been part of human existence. In ancient times we couldn't count on finding food again anytime soon after a big meal, so our bodies evolved to retain energy and store extra calories as fat. What has changed over the past 50,000 years—and especially over the last one hundred years—is that instead of eating 2 cups of leaves as an 80-calorie spinach salad, we can reach for an 8-ounce cup of mini-cookies or a small bag of corn chips and consume 400 to 600 calories in virtually an instant. We also walk less and move less and worry more and eat when we are stressed. Our genes don't have a chance to keep up, since they can only evolve at a rate of ½ percent per million years of evolution.

Principle 4: All Diets Work for Some People

As you'll learn if you spend time at a water cooler in an American office, lots of people lose weight each year and then regain it by following the latest diet fad. Inevitably, they say that a simple change worked for them. The truth is that without major changes in their lifestyles, these dieters regain their lost weight and add more pounds each year. Today, one in two Americans is overweight, with waistlines expanding every day. You can join this large group of dieters who fool themselves into thinking the next quick fix will work, or you can get serious about change. If you change your diet temporarily by eating less sugar, more fat, or simply less food, you will eventually go back to eating "normally." If any so-called diet revolution worked permanently, then we wouldn't need the next season's crop of di-

Principles of Dieting and Your Body Shape

etary fads. However, like a fish in an aquarium, you'll eventually drink the water. Once you go back to the typical American diet of hidden fat, hidden sugar, and too few fruits and vegetables, you will regain your weight. The way to lose weight for good is to change your diet and lifestyle permanently by dealing with what got you here in the first place.

Principle 5: The Real Bottom Line on Protein, Carbs, and Fats

You can fool yourself by thinking that all you need to know is whether a food is a protein, carbohydrate, or fat. There is a lot more to foods than these simple categories. Today food manufacturers can give you any profile you want by messing with Mother Nature. Two foods can have similar proportions of calories, whether or not they contain vitamins, minerals, fiber, and special substances called "phytochemicals" that are necessary for your good health. Simply looking at the protein, carbohydrate, or fat in a food tells you very little about its health-giving qualities. Fortification with vitamins is cheap and doesn't make up for the thousands of phytochemicals found in fruits, vegetables, and whole grains missing from many processed foods. More often than not, processed foods contain added sugar and fat to enhance taste inexpensively. In fact, using clever chemical concoctions, foods can be manipulated to have almost any flavor you can imagine. Dissatisfaction with this state of affairs has led to a whole-foods revolution with natural food sections in markets and special markets entirely devoted to healthier foods.

The Science of Shape: The Belly Fat

Most people think being obese means being really fat. By definition, obesity means having enough excess fat that doctors are willing to agree that you may be putting your health at risk. The fact is that one of two Americans is overweight or obese, and that the overweight tend to become obese over time. The body is more than a container that gets bigger or smaller. Understand your body and how it works, and you can master your metabolism once and for all. First of all, shape is more important than weight. Throughout Asia, which has contributed significantly to the increase in the number of obese and overweight people in the world, the risk of obesity-associated diseases such as heart disease increases at much lower weights than in Americans. The Body Mass Index, or BMI, in Americans is set at 25 for the overweight and 30 for the obese. In Asia, the numbers that give the same increased risk are 23 for the overweight and 27 for the obese. This means that Asians are not gaining weight all over and looking like your typical American couch potato, but rather are gaining it in a spot where it increases the risk of developing heart disease. That spot is the belly or, as we've called it, the apple shape. So you can be at a normal weight, but carry too much fat in the wrong place.

Did you ever wonder why extra fat goes right to your middle? Abdominal fat cells are related to white blood cells—the same cells that protect you from infection. The primary reason that people die from malnutrition is a simple infection, so we have evolved this special tissue that both stores fat and fights infection. It is a great adaptation for a world in which calories are scarce and infections abound. But fighting weight gain, not weight loss, is the battle most of us face as we go through life. These fat cells overdo a good thing by continuing to produce hormones and special proteins called "cytokines" to store fat efficiently, keep your

Principles of Dieting and Your Body Shape

blood sugar up between meals, and stimulate inflammation. Inflammation can help fight infection, which is a good thing if you are malnourished. On the other hand, if you are overweight, then inflammation can be bad. We now know that inflammation is a common denominator for the worst chronic diseases we face today, including heart disease and many common forms of cancer. And the special fat cells in the abdomen also cause a rise in the level of C-reactive protein in the blood, which is an independent risk factor for heart disease.

Belly fat behaves differently than hip or thigh fat, and responds to stress hormones such as cortisol by getting larger. So, the prescription for increasing your belly fat is simply eating more, exercising less, and being stressed out. My goal in this book has been to teach you how to undo this damage and get on the road to a healthier body shape.

Just the Beginning

This is not the end of the L.A. Shape Diet, but rather the beginning. Now that you know how to improve your quality of life through this program of better eating, exercise, and stress reduction, what can you do to stem the rising tide of obesity and its associated diseases, including heart disease and common forms of cancer?

Tell a friend about the ideas in this book. In all my research programs, I have found that the best way to recruit new volunteers for a weight-loss study is through word of mouth. It even beats out television as a way to recruit to research studies. There is a human network out there that is now amplified through the technology of the Internet, so that today it's easier than ever to reach tens of millions of people.

This book is just the beginning of a worldwide movement to improve our bodies by controlling what we eat and how we exercise, and making sure the foods we are sold and our school and job environments make exercise and healthy eating not only possible, but easy.

My goal is to have a world in which everyone loves their personal shape and gets the protein they need each day to control their hunger and keep them from eating the wrong foods. I want a world where instead of being faced with high-fat and high-sugar snacks, you have to *work* to overeat. I want a world where it is harder to be sedentary than it is to be active. I want a world in which everyone makes it a priority to consume the healthy substances found in fruits and vegetables. When that day comes, it will be easier than ever to have both an attractive body shape and protection from premature heart disease and cancer.

But it starts with you. Women suffer especially from being unable to attain the shape they would like in a country where you can never be too thin or too rich. Men largely ignore their expanding waistlines until lower-back or knee pain or even a serious disease wakes them up. Even then many men deny their illnesses, and it is left to their wives to try to care for their health and nutrition.

Serious chronic diseases, such as heart disease and cancer, don't develop overnight. They usually develop over decades. This book is about prevention—changing your health and quality of life now so that you will live longer and better.

Principles of Dieting and Your Body Shape

Appendix

The Science of Meal Replacement

I chuckle when I read the title to this appendix, because "meal replacement" is the term the scientific community gave to diets they rejected as fads just twenty years ago. In the mid-1970s, liquid diets of all kinds were being used—some safe and some unsafe. There are two reasons these diets worked. First, when you are drinking something, you don't think you're eating. So if your hunger is satisfied, you move on through your day without scarfing down burgers and fries for lunch or a Danish pastry and coffee for breakfast. Second, we are well adapted to starvation, so even when eating almost nothing you will still be able to control your physical hunger as your body adapts to eating less food. The comedian Dick Gregory was famous for the fruit juice fasts he used as political protests. He could survive for months on these fasts.

A few years ago, a group of UCLA students camped out in front of the administration building and claimed that they were going to fast and kill themselves in a week if they didn't get what they wanted. They would take only liquids until UCLA agreed to establish a new academic department. I received a call from UCLA's vice chancellor, who asked me if they could go through with their threat. By chance, I was writing a textbook chapter on this topic when he called. I told him that with adequate liquids, vitamins, and minerals they should survive for about six months. This moved the negotiations ahead, and the dispute was soon settled.

Fasting in this way has often been used as a weight-loss treatment over the last century. The late Dr. Ernst Drenick, a UCLA obesity specialist, was featured in a *Life* magazine article in the 1960s about starvation as a treatment for severe obesity. The only problem was that you would lose muscle at a proportion of 1 pound for every 4 pounds of weight you lost with this method.

Protein-modified fasting, also known as very-low-calorie dieting, was developed clinically by Dr. Victor Vertes at the Cleveland Clinic in the late 1970s. In this method, which was validated by the scientific studies of Dr. George Blackburn and Dr. Vernon Young at MIT, the idea was that you could take in enough protein to restore what was being lost. It worked to some extent and was safe as long as people consumed high-quality proteins and had their blood tested every week. The amount of calories in this diet was extremely low, in the range of 375 to 400 calories per day.

Satisfying physical hunger to some extent with a liquid meal was the basis of the Opti-Fast diet, which was provided through hospitals beginning in the late 1970s. In 1977, my close colleague and friend the late Dr. Morton H. Maxwell brought this method of dieting to Los Angeles at the Risk Factor Obesity Clinic, which is still in operation today under my direction at UCLA. This clinic collects data on all the patients enrolled and includes a multidisciplinary team of psychologists, exercise physiologists, nurses, and dietitians who meet weekly. The emotional support provided by this center has led to miraculous results, with patients losing large amounts of weight safely and effectively maintaining their weight loss for years.

In the late 1970s, the very low calorie Cambridge diet was sold to people door-to-door without medical monitoring and caused about eighty deaths around the country, mostly in women with less than 40 pounds to lose. These women lost muscle protein from their hearts, because they had small protein reserves. The massively obese patients did better, because they could draw upon their huge protein reserves. Since the heart is both a muscle and an electrical generator that regulates its own beating, the muscle loss in these women resulted in fatal heart attacks as their hearts stopped beating. Due to this bad publicity, doctors avoided having much to do with these diets, leaving it to specialists like Dr. Maxwell, who developed centers like the one at UCLA to carry on quietly saving thousands of lives over the years.

In the 1970s and 1980s, research probed how these diets worked from a nutritional viewpoint, and this research led ultimately to the development of high carbohydrate/low-fat/low-protein meal replacements that were sold over the counter. This grew to be a huge business. Typically these meal replacements contained between 6 and 8 grams of protein, about 40 grams of sugar, artificial flavorings, vitamins, and minerals. They didn't taste great, but they worked. In 1988, Oprah Winfrey went on the Opti-Fast diet at a Chicago area hospital and lost 65 pounds. In 1989, Tommy Lasorda, the manager of the Los Angeles Dodgers, went on an over-the-counter meal-replacement plan and advertised on television, "If I can do it, you can do it!" He lost 50 pounds, and that year more than thirty million Americans tried meal replacements.

At about this time, I started my research with meal replacements. I had seen the results in my clinic, but in the late 1980s I started to document the effects on blood pressure, cholesterol, and blood sugar in diabetics, and the results were amazing—I was able to reduce or eliminate lots of expensive medications. In 1994, I supervised a study of more than 300 patients at six medical centers in the United States. They were paid $25 a week and given a can of the powdered meal replacement each week. They mixed the powder with milk and drank a shake twice a day for weight loss, together with a reasonable dinner providing about 1,200 calories per day. Again the results were astounding. Men lost 24 pounds in twelve weeks on average. Women lost 12 pounds in twelve weeks, but by twenty-four weeks, both men and women had lost an average of 17 pounds. In 1994, I published these results in a paper entitled, "Clinical evaluation of a minimal intervention meal replacement regimen for weight reduction," in the *Journal of the American College of Nutrition.*

In the late 1990s a series of studies was done that demonstrated the impact of meal replacements on blood pressure, cholesterol, triglycerides, blood sugar, and sleep disorders. Our own unit at UCLA conducted key studies showing that meal replacements were safe and effective when used for type 2 diabetes with obesity (what I call diabesity). In these studies, weight loss with meal replacements led to reduction or elimination of expensive medications used to treat high blood sugar in these diabetic patients after a relatively modest weight loss of about 5 percent of body weight. This amount of weight loss in a study called the Diabetes Prevention Program prevented 58 percent of new cases of diabetes over five years in people who had high blood sugars (but had not yet developed diabetes) and was better at prevention of diabetes than a drug approach.

However, the most striking study was done by Dr. Herwig Ditschuneit at the University of Ulm in Germany. In most American studies, we lose between 20 and 40 percent of participants in research studies by the end of one year. This is not because we lose track of them; studies have shown that volunteers in weight-loss research studies are always looking for the magic bullet and tend to abandon these studies in midstream. Given the strict oversight of Human Subjects Protection Committees at UCLA and elsewhere, it is no longer possible to provide strong monetary incentives linked in any way to continued participation in research. This is now considered unethical, as it is viewed as forcing the patient to participate in the research. We do have to pay for parking and provide the patients with monetary compensation for their participation not linked in any way to attending sessions in the research study. So we can hand out some goodies, such as pedometers, and provide theater tickets and lotteries for gifts, and that's about it.

I bring this up because Dr. Ditschuneit kept 75 percent of his patients on his study for four years and proved that meal replacements were not just effective for weight loss, but also for weight maintenance. He couldn't leave the patients on two meal replacements a day for four years, so the study had an interesting design. For the first twelve weeks, volunteers were randomly assigned either to try to cut down on eating their favorite foods to reach a target of 1,200 calories per day or to follow a meal replacement plan at the same number of calories, which involved drinking two meal replacements a day and eating a healthy dinner. At the end of twelve weeks, the group that tried to cut down on their favorite foods lost a pound or two on average, but the meal replacement group lost 14 pounds. At that point, both groups were told to have one meal replacement a day. By the end of four years, the group that consumed two meal replacements a day for twelve weeks and then one a day for four years lost 10 percent of their body weight. The group that started the meal replacements after twelve weeks and had one per day for four years lost 5 percent. There were also significant changes in some of the risk factors for obesity-associated diseases such as glucose and insulin levels, with larger changes in the group that lost 10 percent of body weight compared to the group that lost 5 percent. A statistician at UCLA analyzed the data, and the results were published in the *American Journal of Clinical Nutrition*.

As a result of all this research, meal replacements are now an accepted method of weight loss treatment. The National Institutes of

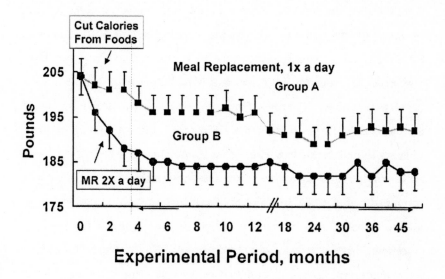

Experimental Period, months

Weight loss over four years using a meal replacement twice a day for twelve weeks (solid triangles) compared to cutting back on favorite foods (solid squares). Until the end of the study at four years, one meal replacement per day was used by both groups (body weight in solid circles). Weight in pounds on the vertical scale is plotted against time in months on the horizontal scale. The figure is adapted from Flechtner-Mors, M., Ditschuneit, H.H., Johnson, T.D., Suchard, M.A., Adler, G. "Metabolic and weight loss effects of long-term dietary intervention in obese patients: four-year results." *Obes Res.* 2000 Aug;8(5):399–402.

The Science of Meal Replacement

Health is sponsoring a multimillion-dollar trial on the effects of weight loss on heart disease in type 2 diabetes patients over five years. Based on some of our research at UCLA and that of others, they have chosen to include meal replacements as a nutritional intervention option in one arm of the study.

However, not all meal replacements are alike. Some taste better than others. The first meal replacements used a lot of sugar and very little protein to optimize taste. Since high-protein diets came into fashion, some have more protein and less sugar but much more fat. When you package a meal replacement in a can, there is a limit to how much protein you can engineer into the liquid without having it settle out. One of the strategies for getting more protein is to add more fat. However, if you have more than 5 grams of fat, your meal replacement is no longer eligible to make any health claims under FDA rules. Some of the high-protein drinks contain 10 grams of fat, which is 90 calories of fat in a 270-calorie high-protein drink. I have designed the Empowering Shake to contain high-quality soy protein and low amounts of fat, and to get its taste from fresh or frozen fruit sugars combined with a moderate amount of carbohydrate. It's impossible to get to zero carbohydrates in a shake, although you will find some meal replacements listing "zero impact carbohydrates." These carbohydrates have fewer short-term effects on blood sugar because of their chemical form, but they are still carbohydrates. As discussed in Step 2, it is important to know that not all carbohydrates are bad; you can review the information on glycemic index, glycemic load, and calories so that you can be smart in picking a healthy meal replacement. Your meal replacement should also have vitamins and minerals or be sold with a companion supplement that provides the vitamins and minerals you need.

I have shown the proof that meal replacements work to hundreds of doctors and dietitians around the country through the North American Association for the Study of Obesity (NAASO) and the Centers for Obesity Research and Education (CORE). NAASO is the leading scientific society on obesity in the country with 1,500 members attending a national and international annual meeting. CORE is a select group of eight obesity research and training programs at university centers of excellence around the country. There are CORE centers at the University of Colorado, UCLA, Harvard Medical School, Columbia University, Northwestern University, Mayo Clinic, University of Minnesota, and the Pennington Biomedical Research Center at Louisiana State University. I am the director of the CORE program at UCLA, with the assistance of Susan Bowerman, who helped me write this book. CORE's mission is to teach primary care doctors and dietitians how to deal with obesity in the setting of the doctor's office. We found that half of all patients being seen in UCLA medical clinics were obese, and that about half would agree to undertake a meal replacement program for weight loss with their doctor's guidance. Unfortunately, as I went around the country with my colleagues trying to convince doctors to take up this challenge, I found that only a minority of them were willing to do so. Weight management doesn't fit the standard medical practice model in this country, and most physicians were just not interested. They were trained to prescribe drugs for the very conditions that weight reduction could help. So I have decided to bring this research on meal replacements directly to you, and to start a movement among ordinary people to use what I have proven scientifically and experienced personally.

References

1. Ashley, J.M., St. Jeor, S.T., Perumean-Chaney, S., Schrage, J., Bovee, V. "Meal replacements in weight intervention." *Obes Res.* 2001 Nov;9 (Suppl 4):312S–320S.

2. Bowerman, S., Bellman, M., Saltsman, P., Garvey, D., Pimstone, K., Skootsky, S., Wang, H.J., Elashoff, R., Heber, D. "Implementation of a primary care physician network obesity management program." *Obes Res.* 2001 Nov;9 (Suppl 4):321S–325S.

3. Flechtner-Mors, M., Ditschuneit, H.H., Johnson, T.D., Suchard, M.A., Adler, G. "Metabolic and weight loss effects of long-term dietary intervention in obese patients: four-year results." *Obes Res.* 2000 Aug;8(5):399–402.

4. Heber, D., Ashley, J.M., Wang, H.J., and Elashoff, R.M. "Clinical evaluation of a minimal intervention meal replacement regimen for weight reduction." *J. Am. Coll. Nutr.* 1994 13:608–14.

5. Hensrud, D.D. "Dietary treatment and long-term weight loss and maintenance in type 2 diabetes." *Obes Res.* 2001 Nov;9 (Suppl 4):348S–353S.

6. Heymsfield, S.B., van Mierlo, C.A., van der Knaap, H.C., Heo, M., Frier, H.I. "Weight management using a meal replacement strategy: meta and pooling analysis from six studies." *Int J Obes Relat Metab Disord.* 2003 May;27(5):537–49.

7. Yip, I., Go, V.L., DeShields, S., Saltsman, P., Bellman, M., Thames, G., Murray, S., Wang, H.J., Elashoff, R., Heber, D. "Liquid meal replacements and glycemic control in obese type 2 diabetes patients." *Obes Res.* 2001 Nov;9 (Suppl 4):341S–347S.

The Science of Protein

This appendix is for those of you who want to learn more about the science behind your personalized protein prescription. How did we arrive at 29 percent of your daily calorie intake, and what is the evidence that protein makes a difference?

There are two kinds of hunger: the psychological kind, which no food can quench, and the physical kind, for which there are biological signals from various types of foods that have been studied scientifically. For every human behavior, including eating, there is both a mind and a body component. Your mind is always capable of overcoming the signals your brain is getting from the body. Nonetheless, if you understand the following mechanisms outlined that make protein work to help you control your cravings, your confidence in the science behind the L.A. Shape Diet may help you lose weight even more effectively.

Protein Is the Most Satisfying

Surviving starvation is just too important for our bodies to depend on any one mechanism or signal pathway. Our best estimates are that at least thirty or forty systems interact in order to prevent starvation, and when one is blocked, another takes over. As a result, I am convinced there will never be a magic pill that you can drop into your serving of french fries in order to lose weight.

But taking in the amount of protein recommended in the L.A. Shape Diet may help to serve this purpose, because it provides a stronger signal to quench your hunger than either carbohydrate or fat over a few hours, over a day, and over months. Protein can also build lean body mass, which increases the number of calories burned per day. Protein is not as efficiently converted into fat as carbohydrate or protein, so when you are trying to maintain your weight it is more difficult to gain weight when you eat more protein. There is a small amount of heat produced (called diet-induced thermogenesis) when you digest your foods and for a short time afterward. Again, protein produces more heat than the same amount of carbohydrate or fat. This heat is energy from the food you eat that is not deposited as fat.

The Amino Acid and Hormone Signals

After a meal, amino acids—the building blocks of protein—are absorbed into the bloodstream, and some cross the blood-brain barrier, where they affect signaling in the brain centers that control hunger. A number of the amino acids, including tryptophan, phenylalanine, and tyrosine, have been theorized to affect the hunger control mechanisms. It is not known exactly how this system works. Some scientists believe that single amino acids enter the brain to reduce hunger while others theorize that some small chains of amino acids survive digestion and are absorbed into the bloodstream and then travel to the brain to help control hunger. Hunger control is a complex matter, and protein intake is likely only one factor—albeit a very important one—in controlling hunger.

Over short periods of time after eating, some proteins are better at satisfying your hunger than others. These are called "fast" proteins, because they release their amino acids into the bloodstream more quickly than other proteins called "slow proteins." Animal proteins also cause slightly more heat production than vegetable proteins. Over the long haul, these small differences become less important; protein is effective in reducing food intake under conditions of free access to food regardless of whether it is animal or vegetable protein.

Researchers in the Netherlands (M.S. Westerterp-Plantenga and co-workers) determined how protein affected hunger perceptions and the body's metabolism in a whole-body energy chamber under controlled conditions for more than 24 hours. Volunteer subjects lived in an enclosed room of about 4 feet by 8 feet; all the air was analyzed for oxygen and carbon dioxide gases, and all food going in and all wastes coming out were carefully measured. In this study, the volunteers were fed exactly the number of calories they burned and were given prescribed exercise and an activity protocol, which was the same on each day. They ate precisely the same amounts of similar foods at identical times in this fully controlled situation. The two diets were a high-protein/high-carbohydrate diet (protein/carbohydrate/fat, percentage of energy 30/60/10) and a high-fat diet (protein/carbohydrate/fat, percentage of energy 10/30/60). Throughout the day, in between meals, subjects reported feeling significantly more satisfied and full on the high-protein/high-carbohydrate diet than on the high-fat diet, while hunger, appetite, desire to eat, and estimated quantity to eat were significantly lower. There was less hunger both during and after the high-protein meals. A higher diet-induced thermogenesis, or heat production, was also observed with the high-protein diet. The amount of the heat produced was directly related to the degree of satisfaction or lack of hunger on the high-protein diet.

Another research team (A.R. Skov and co-workers) compared a high-protein diet with a control diet in order to evaluate weight loss over 27 weeks. Two groups of twenty-five moderately obese volunteers were allowed to eat as much of either of two diets as they wanted. The two diets were 25 percent protein, 45 percent carbohydrate, and 30 percent fat versus 12 percent protein, 58 percent carbohydrate, and 30 percent fat. It was found that weight loss (8.9 versus 5.1 kilograms) and fat loss (7.6 versus 4.3 kilograms) were significantly higher in the higher-protein group, due to about a 16 percent reduction in daily calorie intake. So, given free access to foods, a higher-protein diet is more satisfying than a lower-protein diet and total calorie intake is reduced, leading to better weight loss.

In tests on rats, protein was also shown to be more powerful than carbohydrate for reducing appetite, and the more protein you gave the rats within a certain range of intake, the more it reduced their overall food intake. The animals were more satiated by protein when the proportion was 35 to 50 percent of the total calories in their diet than when the protein was lower and carbohydrate was higher. At least one day was necessary, however, before a significant decrease in calorie intake following the protein loads was observed; thus the animals had somehow to experience the biological effects of the higher protein on their hunger control center for some time before they reduced their food intake. The authors conclude that the larger the proportion of protein in the food, the larger the satiating effect.

Another group (B.J. Brehm and co-workers) studied for six months the effects of a very-low-carbohydrate diet and a calorie-restricted low-fat diet on body weight and heart disease risk factors in healthy women. The very-low-carbohydrate diet group lost more weight (8.5 versus 3.9 kilograms) and more body fat (4.8 versus 2.0 kilograms) than the low-fat group. While this study emphasized that the group with more weight loss was eating a low-carbohydrate diet, they were actually eating significantly more protein than before they started the diet (28 percent versus 16 percent). On the other hand, the low-fat group only increased their intake of protein from 15 percent to 18 percent of total calories on the high-carbohydrate and low-fat diet. So the results may be due to the high-protein levels in that diet rather than what these researchers emphasized as a test of a low-fat diet (actually high carb/low protein) versus a very-low-carbohydrate diet (actually a higher-fat, higher-protein diet). In addition, the group eating more protein, which these researchers called the very-low-carbohydrate group, actually maintained a higher lean body mass while losing weight and a greater percentage of the weight they lost came from excess body fat. So, more protein may help you keep the muscle and lose the fat.

These several studies suggest that body weight loss on a high-protein diet is greater under free-living conditions, in which you can eat as much as you want of the test diet, because less food was eaten on the high-protein diets. In 2002, a review of several different studies of high-protein diets was carried out using a technique called meta-analysis (J. Eisenstein and co-workers). Meta-analysis compares different studies, then combines similar data from these studies in order to examine a scientific question. The advantage is that by pooling all the data you can, you get a more convincing case and an overview of what can be proven on average. The weakness is that studies may have differences in design that limit whether or not you should combine these data into the pool for analysis. To overcome this, the author of a meta-analysis sets up rules for which studies will be considered for pooling. This meta-analysis looking at different studies concluded that, on average, high-protein diets were associated with a 9 percent decrease in total calorie intake. The role of protein in affecting overall calorie intake and in body weight regulation in comparison to fat and carbohydrate still needs more research. But the evidence is strong that protein works, and that your body will feel the difference when you eat more of it. Protein acts on the hunger-signaling mechanisms in the brain, causes more heat generation and calorie burning after it is eaten, and contributes to building lean body mass. For all these reasons, I have recommended that you take in about 29 percent of your total calories from protein.

References

1. Bensaid, A., Tome, D., Gietzen, D., et al. "Protein is more potent than carbohydrate for reducing appetite in rats." *Physiol Behav.* 2002; 75:577–82.

    An elegant study in rats comparing in great detail satiating effects from protein with those from carbohydrates.

2. Bensaid, A., Tome, D., L'Heureux-Bourdon, D., et al. "A high-protein diet enhances satiety without conditioned taste aversion in the rat." *Physiol Behav.* 2003; 78:311–20.

    An important study in rats excluding the suspicion that reduced protein intake may be due to taste aversion.

3. Brehm, B.J., Seeley, R.J., Daniels, S.R., et al. "A randomized trial comparing a very low carbohydrate diet and a calorie-restricted low fat diet on body weight and cardiovascular risk factors in healthy women." *JCEM.* 2003; 88:1617–23.

    An important study that shows the effects from high-protein intake under ad-libitum conditions during a negative energy balance on body weight loss, body composition, as well as the metabolic profile.

4. Billeaud, C., Guillet, J., Sandler, B. "Gastric emptying in infants with or without gastro-oesophageal reflux according to the type of milk." *Eur J Clin Nutr.* 1990; 4:577–83.

5. Boirie, Y., Dangin, M., Gachon, P., et al. "Slow and fast dietary proteins differently modulate postprandial protein accretion." *Proc Nat Acad Sci U S A.* 1997; 94:14930–35.

6. Dulloo, A.G., Jacquet, J. "Low-protein overfeeding: a tool to unmask susceptibility to obesity in humans." *Int J Obes Relat Metab Disord.* 1999; 23:1118–21.

7. Dumesnil, J.G., Turgeon, J., Tremblay, A., et al. "Effect of a low-glycemic index—low-fat—high protein diet on the atherogenic metabolic risk profile of abdominally obese men." *Br J Nutr.* 2001; 86:557–68.

8. Eisenstein, J., Roberts, S.B., Dallal, G., Saltzman, E. "High-protein weight-loss diets: are they safe and do they work? A review of experimental and epidemiologic data." *Nutr Rev.* 2002; 60:189–200.

   A review emphasizing the modulatory effect of dietary protein on energy intake via the sensation of satiety and on energy expenditure by increasing the thermic effect of feeding in short-term studies.

9. Hall, W.L., Millward, D.J., Long, S.J., Morgan, L.M. "Casein and whey exert different effects on plasma amino acid profiles, gastrointestinal hormone secretion and appetite." *Br J Nutr.* 2003; 89:239–48.

   The only study until now dealing with short-term differences in satiety due to different types of protein.

10. Jean, C., Fromentin, G., Tome, D., Larue-Achagiotis, C. "Wistar rats allowed to self-select macronutrients from weaning to maturity choose a high-protein, high-lipid diet." *Physiol Behav.* 2002; 76:65–73.

    A study in rats suggesting that preference for protein may be related to the condition with respect to lean body mass that is present in the animal.

11. Jean, C., Rome, S., Mathe, Y., et al. "Metabolic evidence for adaptation to a high protein diet in rats." *J Nutr.* 2001; 131:91–98.

12. Latner, J.D., Schwartz, M. "The effects of a high-carbohydrate, high protein or balanced lunch upon later food intake and hunger ratings." *Appetite.* 1999; 33:119–28.

13. Laymen, D.K., Boileau, R.A., Erickson, D.J., et al. "A reduced ratio of dietary carbohydrate to protein improves body-composition and blood lipid profiles during weight loss in adult women." *J Nutr.* 2003; 133:411–17.

    This study shows effects from high-protein intake under iso-energetic conditions, emphasizing the metabolic effects of a high-protein diet.

14. Lejeune, M.P.G.M., Kovacs, E.M.R., Westerterp-Plantenga, M.S. "Additional protein intake limits weight regain after weight loss in humans [abstract]." *Int J Obes Relat Metab Disord.* 2003; 27:S25.

15. Mikkelsen, P.B., Toubro, S., Astrup, A. "Effect of fat-reduced diets on 24 h energy expenditure: comparisons between animal protein, vegetable protein, and carbohydrate." *Am J Clin Nutr.* 2000; 72:1135–41.

16. Pullar, J.D., Webster, A.J.F. "The energy cost of fat and protein disposition in the rat." *Br J Nutr.* 1977; 37:355–63.

17.   Raben, A., Agerholm-Larsen, L., Flint, A., et al. "Meals with similar energy densities but rich in protein, fat, carbohydrate, or alcohol have different effects on energy expenditure and substrate metabolism but not on appetite and energy intake." *Am J Clin Nutr.* 2003; 77:91–100.

An elaborate study comparing appetite as well as energy metabolism effects of all different macronutrients at the same time.

18.   Skov, A.R., Toubro, S., Ronn, B., et al. "Randomized trial on protein vs. carbohydrate in ad libitum fat reduced diet for the treatment of obesity." *Int J Obes Relat Metab Disord.* 1999; 23:528–36.

19.   Stock, M.J. "Gluttony and thermogenesis revisited." *Int J Obes Relat Metab Disord.* 1999; 23:1105–17.

The author of the Stock Hypothesis, which states that protein reduces hunger because of its greater effects on thermogenesis.

20.   Westerterp-Plantenga, M.S., Lejeune, M.P.G.M., Nijs, I., et al. "High protein intake sustains weight maintenance after body weight loss in humans [abstract]." *Int J Obes Relat Metab Disord.* 2003; 27:S127.

21.   Westerterp-Plantenga, M.S., Rolland, V., Wilson, S.A.J., Westerterp, K.R. "Satiety related to 24 h diet-induced thermogenesis during high protein/carbohydrate vs. high fat diets measured in a respiration chamber." *Eur J Clin Nutr.* 1999; 53:495–502.

22.   Westerterp-Plantenga, M.S., Westerterp, K.R., Rubbens, M., et al. "Appetite at 'high altitude,' operation Everest-Comex: a simulated ascent of Mt. Everest." *J Appl Physiol.* 1999; 87:391–99.

The Science of Shape and Body Fat

Your body fat actually takes the form of several vital organs, just like your heart, liver, kidney, or skin. These organs contain nerves, blood vessels, and fat cells, and they secrete hormones and proteins that affect energy balance, fat storage, and metabolism. The function of the body fat organs depends on where they are located on your body. Each of the body fat organs in the lower body (for women) and in the upper body (for both men and women) have special functions with regard to the uptake and release of fatty acids and in terms of the hormones they secrete and to which they respond. In the 1990s, it was found that fat cells secrete a small hormone called "leptin" that binds to receptors in the brain to reduce food intake and increase physical activity. There is emerging evidence that leptin comes from both lower- and upper-body fat, whereas another fat cell–produced protein, adiponectin, comes largely from the abdominal fat and affects blood clotting, which is part of your immune defense system. So, the science of shape and the science of how your body fat communicates with other organs and the brain are all connected. I will try to summarize this rapidly changing area, but you will need to keep up on your own as the science is moving quickly.

Female Fat

The fat on women's hips and thighs supplies the energy mothers need to provide milk for their newborn babies. This fat responds to female hormones, and in every menstrual cycle, right after ovulation, there is a 1,000-fold increase in the blood levels of the female hormone progesterone. When women believe they are gaining small amounts of weight in addition to being bloated, they are right. The body is preparing for pregnancy by developing the fat organs in the hips and thighs—and if a woman becomes pregnant, they will grow much more, due to the large amounts of estrogen and progesterone produced by the placenta. A considerable number of calories must be stored, since breast milk production normally requires about 500 calories per day.

The main factor accounting for female obesity is weight gain after pregnancy. Women typically gain between 30 and 40 pounds during pregnancy. If they do not breast feed or diet and exercise in the six months after delivery, the weight gained during pregnancy is typically not lost. The next pregnancy starts at a higher weight, and more weight is gained with the second pregnancy—and so forth. Understanding how this fat accumulates can help young women lose weight after delivering their children and can lead to prevention of obesity.

Just as women are born with different-shaped bodies, they're born with different-sized hip and thigh fat organs. There is nothing wrong with that kind of fat, except that our modern society has labeled it bad. Historically, women with fat in their lower bodies were always in demand, and biology reflected what was desirable. There is a disconnect between women's genetics and what is considered attractive by many people today. However, there is a backlash. Jennifer Lopez has come out with a line of lingerie "in large sizes," and African-American women and men have definitely spoken out about the attractiveness of larger women. One of my key messages is that there needs to be more tolerance of different body shapes in our society.

This fat does tend to be more resistant to diet and exercise, and many women starve themselves trying to lose it. In the pursuit of skinnier thighs, some even lose an unhealthy amount of fat in their faces and chests. It is important to be aware of your appropriate target weight and shape if you have more fat in the hips and thighs than in the upper body.

Abdominal Fat

The fat in the middle of the body surrounds the intestines and has special properties both in terms of the substances it releases into the bloodstream and in the hormones to which it responds. Both men and women can accumulate abdominal fat. There are women who have mainly upper-body fat and never accumulate much lower-body fat, and there are also women who accumulate both upper- and lower-body fat.

Women with upper-body fat have higher male hormone levels than women with lower-body fat. They are three times more likely to get breast cancer and about nine times more likely to get diabetes than women with predominantly lower-body fat.

Upper-body fat is designed to enable you to survive starvation. It secretes a number of substances called "cytokines" that fight infection. In fact, this protection from infection is a key function of upper-body fat that is part of the adaptation of mankind to starvation or famine. One of the major causes of death from starvation is infection, and your upper-body fat protects you from this complication of malnutrition.

This fat also responds to the stress hormone cortisol, which comes from the adrenal gland. (In army helicopter pilots, cortisol levels in the blood have been shown to rise tenfold in wartime.) In a disease called "Cushing's syndrome," there is overproduction of cortisol by the adrenal glands, with a resulting increase in this fat organ in the middle of the body. There is an enzyme, 11-betahydroxysteroid dehydrogenase, that can convert cortisone to cortisol. Mice that are genetically altered to produce more of this enzyme accumulate fat only in the abdomen and not in other fat organs.

Abdominal fat is easier to lose with dieting than lower-body fat. It is often the first fat to be lost in those who have both upper- and lower-body fat. However, with stress it is easy to gain this weight back quickly. I recently saw two patients in the same day who gained 13 pounds in a month due to increased stress and an inability to stay on their diet plan. So-called yo-yo dieters often have upper-body fat.

Brain Centers and Body Fat

The fat cells make leptin, a hormone named for the Greek word for thinning. It was first discovered in a mutant line of obese mice that made a defective version of this hormone. These mice develop about 60 percent of their body weight as fat tissue. When normal mice had their circulation merged with these obese mice, they corrected the abnormality, and the mice lost weight.

Leptin is sensed in a part of the brain called the "Arcuate nucleus" of the hypothalamus, where it is one of many different signals to the brain. Leptin deficiency is extremely rare, but there is a village in Turkey where a family has this deficiency. My colleague Dr. Julio Licinio at UCLA recently treated this family with leptin, and they lost huge amounts of weight, going from massively obese to a normal size. Leptin has other effects, too; it reduces food intake and increases physical activity. It also inhibits new blood vessel formation, and this is another way it may inhibit new fat tissue growth in the genetically obese mouse.

Insulin, the feeding hormone that is produced by the pancreas, goes up after eating. It pushes fats into fat cells for storage and amino acids into muscle, and it stores some sugars as starch in the liver and muscle. Insulin and leptin both rise in response to nutrients such as glucose and amino acids. For the last thirty years, Dr. Daniel Porte, now at the University of California, San Diego, has championed the theory that obesity is due to a lack of normal insulin action in the brain. He has demonstrated in primate studies that high levels of insulin in the blood are associated with reduced insulin action in the brain.

Leptin levels change in the opposite direction to another peptide, neuropeptide Y, or NPY. When leptin goes down, NPY increases in the brain. NPY has the opposite effect of leptin, and it increases food intake. So the body builds in hormones that work in both directions, and I believe we have only scratched the surface of this control system that maintains body weight, food intake, and physical activity in the brain. Recently another hormone was discovered in the brain that reduces food intake and was named "orexin."

In addition to the hormones made by fat cells and those found in the brain, there is a hormone called "ghrelin" that is made by stomach cells. Its strange name comes from its ability to release growth hormone (gh) from the pituitary gland. Ghrelin blood levels go up between meals, stimulating appetite. Obese individuals have higher rises of ghrelin between meals. Obese individuals who have stomach bypass surgery experience a decrease in appetite after their operations, and their levels of ghrelin fall below detectable concentrations.

Further down the gastrointestinal tract in the small intestine are the glucagon like peptides (GLPs), which are released from the intestine and affect food intake. Cholecystokinin is a hormone named for its ability to contract the gallbladder, which usually happens after a high-fat meal. A form of this hormone is believed to be transported into the brain as well to control food intake. As if this were not enough, fat tissue makes other hormones, including omentin, vasofatin, and resistin, that have effects on the breakdown of nutrients by the body. Some of the hormones made in abdominal fat are not secreted into the bloodstream, but work within the abdominal fat organ to regulate its activity and what it secretes into the bloodstream that affects food intake, metabolism, and physical activity. In short, maintaining body weight in the face of starvation is a very important and basic bodily function that is maintained by overlapping groups of hormones produced all over the body, but the fat organs have a lot to do with transmitting to the brain the state of your nourishment.

Genes and Obesity

Obesity is the result of an interaction of genes and environment. There are currently about seventeen different genes that we know can account for obesity. Nonetheless, the total number of individuals with these genetic diseases account for only 5 percent of all cases of obesity. Some of these disorders are fascinating and involve multiple problems in mental functioning, reproduction, vision, and facial appearance. However, the majority of the obese population is simply well adapted to starvation. Research on the genes involved in familial obesity have so far shown up some seventy associations with parts of the human genome. These studies merely map parts of the genetic material where important genes may exist, and these many associations simply point out again how serious the body is about regulation of food intake and body weight. However, it is unlikely that any of these search methods will uncover any unique targets that account for a significant percentage of obesity cases. Rather, most experts suggest any one defect may contribute about 2 percent to the tendency to gain weight. Somehow the cumulative effects of multiple genes are what tip the balance toward gaining weight.

On the other hand, it is the sedentary lifestyle of the current age that combines with the high-fat, high-sugar, and high-starch diet to unmask the genes for obesity. It is generally believed that the very obese people more than 100 pounds overweight or with a BMI higher than 40 have the greatest genetic programming for obesity. In the last ten years, the overall rate of obesity (BMI>40) has doubled in this country, and the number of people with severe obesity (BMI>40) has increased fourfold, according to a recent Rand study.

However, beyond obesity in general, your shape is genetic. Identical twins reared apart not only have similar body weights, but photographs of their fat distribution show almost identical pockets of fat. So, your body's shape is genetically determined, but it can be altered with diet and lifestyle changes.

The Bottom Line

The key message here is that your shape reflects your particular pattern of fat deposits. These can be altered with diet and lifestyle changes, as discussed elsewhere in this book. However, there are enough complex controls on body fat and a communication between fat tissue and brain to make it impossible to fool Mother Nature beyond a certain point. Selecting a realistic shape and target weight goal is essential to succeeding on this or any program.

References

1. Asakawa, A., Inui, A., Yuzuriha, H., Ueno, N., Katsuura, G., Fujimiya, M., Fujino, M.A., Niijima, A., Meguid, M.M., Kasuga, M. "Characterization of the effects of pancreatic polypeptide in the regulation of energy balance." *Gastroenterology.* 2003 May; 124(5):1325–36.

2. Bombard, Y. "Do these genes make me look fat? Obesity and melanocortin-4 receptor gene deficiencies." *Clin Genet.* 2003 Nov;64(5):380–81.

3. Challis, B.G., Pinnock, S.B., Coll, A.P., Carter, R.N., Dickson, S.L., O'Rahilly, S. "Acute effects of PYY(3–36) on food intake and hypothalamic neuropeptide expression in the mouse." *Biochem Biophys Res Commun.* 2003 Nov; 28;311(4):915–19.

4. Herzog, H. "Neuropeptide Y and energy homeostasis: insights from Y receptor knockout models." *Eur J Pharmacol.* 2003 Nov; 7;480(1–3): 21–9.

5. Nagasawa, A., Fukui, K., Kojima, M., Kishida, K., Maeda, N., Nagaretani, H., Hibuse, T., Nishizawa, H., Kihara, S., Waki, M., Takamatsu, K., Funahashi, T., Matsuzawa, Y. "Divergent effects of soy protein diet on the expression of adipocytokines." *Biochem Biophys Res Commun.* 2003 Nov; 28;311(4):909–14.

6. Ouchi, N., Kihara, S., Funahashi, T., Matsuzawa, Y., Walsh, K. "Obesity, adiponectin and vascular inflammatory disease." *Curr Opin Lipidol.* 2003 Dec;14(6):561–66.

7. Paoloni-Giacobino, A., Grimble, R., Pichard, C. "Genomic interactions with disease and nutrition." *Clin Nutr.* 2003 Dec;22(6):507–14.

8. Perusse, L., Bouchard, C. "Genetics of obesity and metabolic complications in the Quebec Family Study." *Med Sci* (Paris). 2003 Oct;19(10):937–42.

9. Silha J.V., Krsek, M., Skrha, J.V., Sucharda, P., Nyomba, B.L., Murphy, L.J. "Plasma resistin, adiponectin and leptin levels in lean and obese subjects: correlations with insulin resistance." *Eur J Endocrinol*. 2003 Oct;149(4):331–35.

10. Staiger, H., Tschritter, O., Machann, J., Thamer, C., Fritsche, A., Maerker, E., Schick, F., Haring, H.U., Stumvoll, M. "Relationship of serum adiponectin and leptin concentrations with body fat distribution in humans." *Obes Res*. 2003 Mar;11(3):368–72.

The Science of Bioimpedance Analysis

Obesity is defined as excess body fat, and ideally the amount of that body fat should be measured scientifically. This can be done by many methods, but none of them is exact. Bioimpedance analysis is the one practical method of body composition analysis that gives you the most useful and scientifically valid information about lean body mass and the number of calories you burn each day. The percent body fat you obtain from this method is an estimate; it will provide you only with a range of healthy body fats related to a range of your personal body shape. You may not care about body fat percentage, but you do care about your dress size or the size of your waist. Ultimately, you'll have to look in the mirror to know whether you are satisfied and are being realistic based on the range of body weights and body fats that you can possibly have and remain healthy.

The percent body fat shows what your ideal shape can be, within a healthy range of body fat (about 22 to 28 percent for women and 15 to 20 percent for men). Athletes have much lower percent body fats, because they have much more muscle mass than average individuals. For example, Magic Johnson, the famous Laker basketball player, wrote in the *Los*

Angeles Times that at 14 percent body fat he felt too fat to play well. He gave up eating nachos with cheese after every game, and his body fat decreased to 4 percent. He felt better, and his game improved. His only worry was that there might be a nachos advisory board that would be angry with him.

In this section I discuss the various methods of measuring body composition and why I believe bioelectrical impedance analysis is the best and most practical way to learn more about your shape.

Underwater Weighing

Since fat floats on water, your body weight underwater is less than it is on land. If I submerge a swing seat underwater and attach it to a scale overhead, I can weigh you both underwater and on land and calculate your percent body fat. The only problem is that the air in your lungs will also make you float, so I can ask you to blow out all the air from your lungs before going underwater. This is a rather unnatural and uncomfortable thing to do, since people generally hold their breath before going underwater. And even if you do try to blow out all the air, there will still be some left in your lungs. This is called "the residual volume." So, if I want to make this method work scientifically, I also have to measure how much air is in your lungs by having you breathe in nitrogen gas, which I sample to determine the volume of air in your lungs.

This method is not practical because I have to get you to wear a bathing suit and find a pool. Once you add up all the potential errors in the various measurements, this method is not the gold standard it is held up to be, so for me it is not worth the trouble. One reason underwater weighing is so loved is that many university physical education and kinesiology departments have invested in water tanks devoted to this method and used it in their research papers.

Another version of underwater weighing is done on land using something called a "Bod Pod." This was developed with federal funding at the University of California at Davis. It is an egg-shaped plastic chamber with a transparent front shell that opens, allowing you to sit on a seat inside. Once the door is closed, the amount of air that your body displaces and your weight on the chair are registered. For those of you who remember high school chemistry, all you need to calculate the density of an object is its volume and weight. This sounds good, but the method requires you to put on a bathing suit. Heavy clothes will displace air just as your body would and will make the measurement less accurate. My patients aren't going to get into a bathing suit in a clinic. My patients find it hard enough to come on a first visit to a doctor whom they don't know without having to go through an embarrassing procedure with his or her staff. In fact, many of my patients won't go swimming until they are happy with their shape and getting into a bathing suit while they are fat would definitely be emotionally traumatic for them.

Tritium Dilution and Total Body Potassium

These methods use radiation to determine percent body fat and are strictly used for research, since giving radioactive substances would be unacceptable on a routine basis.

Tritium is a radioactive form of hydrogen that can be found naturally in water. It is produced industrially for medical research by concentrating large volumes of water. My first job as a college sophomore at UCLA was working for the Nobel Prize winner Dr. Willard F. Libby, who discovered radiocarbon dating. My job was to run a huge cooler with a battery in it that evaporated water slowly. I was responsible for evaporating huge volumes of water to produce tritium. All water has two hydrogen atoms and one oxygen atom (H_2O), but in tritium the hydrogen atoms are radioactive. If I weigh a syringe full of this radioactive water and inject it into your bloodstream, I can collect blood samples over the next few hours, and the radioactivity will be decreased by an amount dependent on the size of your body water pool which is for all intents and purposes nonradioactive.

Imagine throwing some ink into both your swimming pool and a smaller pool at your neighbor's house. If you threw in the same amount of ink and then took a sample of the water, whoever had the larger pool would have less of the ink color in the pool water. Once I know the amount of water in your body, I can subtract from your body weight and get an estimate of the amount of fat in your body.

The total body potassium method is only available in a few places in the world (one being UCLA). It involves having you sit in a leather sling chair with a large crystal placed a few feet away and hovering over your stomach. You sit in the chair for 45 minutes, and the natural radiation from potassium in your body is measured on the crystal. As the potassium releases its natural radioactivity, the energy is absorbed by the crystal and an electrical signal is generated in the crystal and recorded on a machine. The more muscle you have, the more potassium there is in your body to release naturally occurring radioactivity. This method requires you to be locked into a steel chamber made out of pre–World War II battleship steel, because once atomic testing began after the war the environment was contaminated with radioactive potassium at such high levels that newer steel would interfere with the machine's ability to detect the radioactive potassium in your body. There is a television camera in the chamber so that a researcher can observe you in case you get claustrophobic and want to climb out before the 45 minutes are up.

Once I know your body potassium, I can calculate your lean body mass, because muscle cells and other organ cells, such as those in the liver, are loaded with potassium. If you visualize yourself sitting in a sling-type hammock leather chair with this crystal trying to catch the radioactivity from your muscles, you will understand the key limitation of this approach. Fat reduces the ability of radioactivity to escape from the body so that it can be detected by the crystal. Therefore, individuals with more abdominal fat will not have as accurate a reading of their lean body mass. While thigh fat will interfere less with radiation from the hips and thighs, there is still a difference in the efficiency of the machine in different people.

DEXA (Dual Energy X-ray Absorptiometry)

The DEXA method uses X rays to estimate body fat and lean. The DEXA machine was originally designed to measure bone density, but its computer can estimate body fat and lean by taking advantage of the different abilities of muscle and fat to block the X rays to give you an image of your body shape and the muscle and fat inside of it. A computer can then calculate the amounts of fat in various regions of the body. We have one of these machines at the UCLA Center for Human Nutrition and have compared its results to those from bioelectrical impedance. DEXA provides a useful answer once you adjust the numbers for research studies. The main drawbacks for using this method for obesity prevention and treatment widely are the expense of the DEXA machine, the 15 minutes it takes (which is more than bioelectrical impedance analysis), and the radiation exposure, which is equal to that given in an abdominal X ray.

Bioelectrical Impedance Analysis

This method depends on the fact that lean tissue is about 70 percent water and conducts electricity, but fat is an insulator that has no water and conducts electricity very poorly. The method can be done in many ways, but only one is valid scientifically.

In the correct method, the researcher uses four electrodes—the same sticky 1-inch squares that doctors use to do electrocardiograms. A black and a red electrode are placed on one of your hands and also on the foot that is on the same side as your hand. A very small alternating electrical current (so small you can't feel it) is passed through your body; the current flows from one red clip to another and from one black clip to another. A meter inside the machine measures an electrical property called "impedance," which is how hard it is for the electrical current to travel between the electrodes. The machine knows the distance between the electrodes based on your height.

This measurement takes only a minute or two once the electrodes are properly attached, and the machine I use displays your percent body fat, lean body mass, and estimated calories burned per day. I push another button, and out comes the target weight, based on a desirable percent body fat. I have used this machine in thousands of patients, and the model I have can be calibrated periodically so that I know it is giving me the correct readings.

Since the machine measures the electrical properties of water in your body, it can be thrown off if you drink too much water before the measurement, or if you have a disease that makes you retain water. It will measure that water as lean body mass. It's also necessary to swab the skin on your hand and foot carefully so that no lotion, sweat, or dirt can interfere with the flow of electricity to your skin. And the electrodes must be placed as in the following diagram; placing them too close together can throw off the measurement by a few percent.

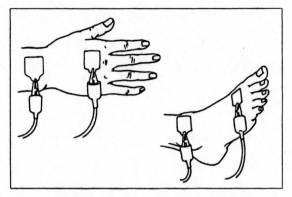

Red clips to the pads near the wrist and ankle joint

Black clips to the pads on the hand and foot

Proper attachment of electrodes for bioelectrical impedance analysis

While this seems like a lot of trouble to go to, it's less trouble than a lot of methods, and it is the only method I use. Department stores sell machines that have you stand on metal electrodes. These machines usually cost under $100, but they pass an electrical current only up to your calves to about your knees. This is not accurate unless you have an average body build. Another kind of machine has metal handles that you grab, and the electrical current only goes up the arms. This one costs about $50 and doesn't give an accurate measure of body fat for the same reason that standing on a meter doesn't work. I saw the most ridiculous fat-measuring machine recently in a store for $15: You place your thumbs on the tiny machine.

How do all of these devices claim to work? They use a mathematical formula based on height and weight, which is the basis of the Body Mass Index (BMI) to estimate body fat (the formula is shown on page 263). The problem is that the formula works for studying average body composition but not for your personal shape. So, these little devices do get lucky once in a while.

When I was demonstrating the bioelectrical impedance method at a health fair, one fellow objected. He noticed that using the thumb device he got as close to the same measure as with the analyzer I was using. I simply passed his thumb device around the room, and it was pretty obvious that for people who were not average-shaped, these other machines don't agree with the four electrode bioimpedance analyzer that I have used and studied in thousands of patients over the past twenty years.

Using Body Mass Index to Estimate Body Fat

Garrow and Webster, two British scientists, did a study that measured body fat, height, and weight in large numbers of research subjects, and in 1985 they wrote a paper that established the Body Mass Index as height divided by the weight squared. This formula is approximate, but it works when averaged over large numbers of people, because most big people in the U.S. have too much body fat on average. However, their paper recognized that the formula was not suitable for use in athletes or the elderly, where the lean body mass is not average. All the football players on the offensive and defensive lines of your favorite college team would be classified as obese, based on their BMIs. However, their weight is mostly due to extra muscle, not fat. Elderly people usually have muscle wasting, so their weight includes more fat.

At UCLA, I found that when I used bioelectrical impedance, a lot of men and women had more muscle than would be expected on average. Their target weights on the machine were 20 or 30 pounds higher than what would be predicted for the average person. Then I measured the body fat of women who looked thin and healthy, and found that these percentages were surprisingly high.

In twenty-eight women between the ages of twenty-four and forty-nine seen in our high-risk breast cancer clinic, I found an average percent body fat of 35 percent, even though the average Body Mass Index was only 23. Their BMIs ranged between 17 and 28, so none of these women were obese by BMI standards (a BMI over 30 is considered obese), but their percent body fat ranged between 25 and 45 percent.

I then measured 306 patients in my weight loss clinic and compared the amount of body fat and lean that would be estimated from their Body Mass Index, drawn from a calculation using height and weight, to what was actually measured by the bioimpedance machine using its internal mathematical equations and the information on the electrical measurement. There are actually equations used to estimate average fat mass from just height in meters and BMI. In case you want to try these equations out on your calculator, here they are:

$$\text{For women: Fat in kilograms} = (0.713 \text{ BMI}—9.74) \text{ Ht}^2$$
$$\text{For men: Fat in kilograms} = (0.715 \text{ BMI}—12.1) \text{ Ht}^2$$

Be sure to convert height into meters. Multiply height in inches by 0.254 to get height in meters. Then multiply the answer by itself to get height in meters squared (Ht^2).

Using these estimates and doing some statistical analyses, I found that the patients could be divided into three groups of about equal size.

- I coined the term "sarcopenic obesity" to describe the condition of the group that looked thin but was actually overfat (like the women in the breast clinic). Sarcopenia means loss of muscle; this term had been applied to the elderly, but not to obese people.

- I used the term "proportionate obesity" to describe the group whose body fat had been perfectly predicted because their bodies had an average shape.

- The third group had more muscle development, or hypermuscular obesity.

The mathematics showed that these groups were really different, and I presented these findings at a meeting held at the National Institutes of Health on Methods of Body Composition. In 1996, I published a paper entitled "Clinical detection of sarcopenic obesity by bioelectrical impedance analysis" in the *American Journal of Clinical Nutrition*. I have referenced that paper at the end of this Appendix section so that you can look it up and examine the scientific evidence on which I base my use of bioelectrical impedance analysis in this book to predict lean body mass, energy needs, and protein requirements in the diet.

Strengths and Limitations of the Bioelectrical Impedance Analysis

Some scientists say that this method doesn't tell them anything more than what they get from height and weight. In large numbers of people averaged out, this is true. However, in any single person who is not average (and you may not be average), I find this machine helps me a lot as I counsel patients using the concepts in this book. I don't repeat the method over and over again on a weekly basis. You can actually have a slight increase in body fat percentage early on in the diet, when you've lost the initial water weight, but before you've lost much fat. Instead, I use it at the beginning to determine the target weight and at some milestone to see how you are doing in reaching your target weight. In our Risk Factor Obesity Clinic at UCLA, we measure patients every twelve weeks. In a group of several hundred severely obese patients at UCLA who lost on average over 120 pounds after a Roux-en-Y gastric bypass surgery for obesity, my colleagues and I were able to predict final weight a year later with a single measurement before surgery.

I have taken the bioelectrical impedance analyzer to various talks in front of small groups, and it is always amazing how people react to their personal information. This is the real strength of this machine. Knowing your cholesterol, blood pressure, and body fat can really make a difference to you personally, especially when that information is used to customize your diet in terms of protein and calories.

References

1. Drenick, E.J., Blahd, W.J., Singer, F.R., Lederer, M. "Body potassium content in obese subjects and potassium depletion during prolonged fasting." *Am J Clin Nutr.* 1966;18:278–85.

2. Garrow, J.S., Webster, J. "Quetelet's Index as a measure of fatness." *Int J Obes Relat Metab Disord.* 1985;9:147–55.

3. Heber, D., Ingles, S., Ashley, J.M., Maxwell, M.H., Lyons, R.F., and Elashoff, R.M. "Clinical detection of sarcopenic obesity by bioelectrical impedance analysis." *Am J Clin Nutr.* 1996;64:472S–477S.

4. Lukaski, H.C., Bolonchuk, W.W., Hall,C.B., Sider, W.A. "Validation of a tetrapolar bioelectrical impedance method to assess human body composition." *J Appl Physiol.* 1986;60:1327–32.

The Science of Good Fats and Bad Fats

I am often asked about which fats are best to eat. For many years, you were told that all fat was bad. Now you are hearing about good fats and bad fats, and that you should substitute healthy fats for unhealthy fats. I think this is great, but which fats and how much of them? I believe you should use just enough fats and oils in your foods to provide great taste, which can be accomplished with about 20 percent of total calories from fat. But when the oil starts dripping off the plate, you're eating too much, no matter how "good" the fat is. All fats have more than 120 calories per tablespoon, and that adds up fast when you are trying to lose weight.

Different Fats and Fatty Acids

The different types of fats and oils in the following list are called "saturated," "monounsaturated," and "polyunsaturated" based on the predominant type of fatty acid, which is the building block of the particular fat or oil.

COMPARISON OF DIETARY FATS AND OILS

Dietary Fat	Saturated Fat	Linoleic Acid	Alpha-Linolenicn Acid	Monounsaturated Fat
Olive Oil	14%	8%	1%	77%
Avocado Oil	15%	11%	1%	62%
Corn Oil	13%	61%	1%	25%
Soybean Oil	15%	54%	7%	24%
Peanut Oil	18%	34%	0%	48%
Safflower Oil	9%	78%	trace	13%
Sunflower Oil	11%	69%	0%	20%
Palm Oil	51%	10%	0%	39%
Lard	41%	11%	1%	47%
Beef Tallow	52%	3%	1%	44%
Butterfat	66%	2%	2%	30%
Coconut Oil	92%	2%	0%	6%

Reference: Agricultural Handbook No.8-4 and Human Nutrition Information Service, USDA, 1979, and California Avocado Commission website nutrition label information, 2003.

In fact, almost all the fat in your diet and in your body is made up of triglycerides. Triglycerides are made up of three fatty acids linked together by a sugar called "glycerol," which is made up of three carbon atoms to which the fatty acids are linked. The fatty acids themselves are long chains of carbon atoms linked by chemical bonds of two main types: a single bond and a double bond. The double bond is made up of electron clouds, which make the bond between the carbons flexible. So, saturated fats are stiff and tend to be solid at room temperature, since the carbon atoms have less flexibility to move than carbons connected by a double bond or electron cloud. Both polyunsaturated fats and monounsaturated fats are liquid oils at room temperature because they are made up of flexible chains of carbons

The Science of Good Fats and Bad Fats

between 18 and 22 carbons long. These chains of carbon atoms bend easily at the one to three places where the double-bond electron clouds occur.

Why Saturation Matters

These physical characteristics of being flexible or stiff translate into lots of different properties for different fats. The solid fats tend to hold flavor and heat better and generally can be heated to higher temperatures. This last property is why lard was used to deep-fry the original fast-food french fry at McDonald's in the 1950s. They later switched to hydrogenated soybean oil, which starts out polyunsaturated and has the double bonds chemically changed to single bonds by a reaction with hydrogen. These chemically altered fats are called "trans-fats" because when they are chemically altered, even though they still have one double bond, it is in an unnatural configuration, so that it acts like a single bond in a saturated fat.

It is pretty much agreed that saturated fats and trans-fats both tend to raise cholesterol levels, and higher levels of cholesterol are a major risk factor for heart disease. In population studies going back to the 1960s and 1970s, blood cholesterol levels have been related to the amount of saturated fat in the diet. As with all population studies, part of this effect is chemical and part is accounted for by saturated fats from meats, denoting a particular dietary and lifestyle pattern associated with other risk factors, such as obesity, that also increase the risk of heart disease.

Read the labels of processed foods and you will see that lots of them contain 50 percent fat calories, often from hydrogenated fats. Hydrogenated fats act like lard or palm oil (both saturated fats) in their ability to hold flavor and heat in foods. Many baked goods require these types of fats in order to bake properly or to maintain the consistency of frosting. This is one reason that pastries, cakes, and muffins appear on my Trigger Foods list. Some companies have removed the trans-fats from snack foods such as potato chips and corn chips when it does not affect flavor.

The government has changed the official nutrition label to include trans-fats. This is largely because of the efforts of Dr. Walter Willett, at the Harvard School of Public Health, who did studies in large populations that demonstrated the connection between trans-fats and heart disease. These studies did not prove that trans-fats cause heart disease, but at the very least they are markers of a diet made up of too many processed foods and too few fruits and vegetables.

The Chemistry of Polyunsaturated Fats

Polyunsaturated fats are also good or bad, depending on where the double bonds occur. The omega-6 fats are more inflammatory, and some call these "bad fats." In omega-6 fats, the first double bond occurs 6 carbons from one end of the chain. The most common fatty acid in corn oil is linoleic acid, which is 18 carbons long and has two double bonds, with the first one 6 carbons from one end of the long carbon chain. Omega-3 fats from fish oil and from plants are called "good fats" because they are anti-inflammatory and counteract the effects of omega-6 fats inside cells. Linoleic acid is the omega-6 fat that we need to eat in small amounts as an essential fat (we don't make it in our bodies), while another 18-carbon fatty acid, linolenic acid, is the essential omega-3 fatty acid. Linolenic acid has three bonds, and the first one is 3 carbons from one end. Since the names sound so similar for linoleic (omega-6) and linolenic (omega-3), scientists use a number system for these two, which are 18:2 n-6 and 18:3 n-3, respectively. The notation means 18 carbons, with either two or three double bonds, and the n-6 or n-3 means that the first double bond is 6 or 3 carbons from one end of this 18-carbon fatty acid.

Fatty Acid Requirements in the Diet

Linoleic acid and linolenic acid are essential elements in the diet. You need to get about 5 percent of your total calories from these fatty acids, which are found in plants. Ancient diets were so rich in plants that over time our bodies gave up making these fatty acids, much as we gave up the genetic machinery for making vitamin C.

You don't need to worry about not getting enough fatty acids in your diet, since plants contain about 10 percent fat and both linoleic and linolenic acids, in a ratio of about three to one. Our modern diets use a lot of processed oils, and the oil manufacturers have stripped out much of the omega-3 fatty acids found naturally in plant oils to clarify them and extend their shelf life in the store. The result is that our modern diet has a ratio of omega-6 to omega-3 fatty acids in the range of between 10 to 1 and 30 to 1, depending on your diet. The ratios include both linoleic and linolenic acids as well as other common omega-6 and omega-3 fatty acids I have not discussed, including omega-3 fish oils eicosapentanoic acid (20:5 n-3) and docosahexanoic acid (22:6 n-3). These are the most famous fatty acids in this class. To know more, you can consult a biochemistry textbook for the most common fatty acids found in humans. My laboratory measures over twenty common fatty acids in the blood, many of which are affected by our diet, while others are made by our bodies. We tend to make saturated fats similar to that found in steaks. I used to show a humorous cartoon where two sharks are circling a human and the caption reads, "Let's pass him up, he's too high in saturated fat."

Ratios and Inflammation

The ratio of omega-6 to omega-3 is sensed by cells throughout the body. Enzymes called "cyclooxygenase enzymes" convert these fatty acids into signals called "eicosanoids." These eicosanoids are small molecules that can either cause inflammation or inhibit inflammation signals in cells. The same enzyme can make both pro-inflammatory and anti-inflammatory signals from omega-6 or omega-3 fatty acids, respectively. Research shows that the ratio of omega-6 to omega-3 fatty acids is one determinant of how much inflammation exists throughout the body. Inflammation is being recognized as a common disease-causing mechanism that is at the root of heart disease, asthma, and many common forms of cancer. When these fatty acids occur in plants, they are eaten together with naturally occurring vitamin E and other antioxidants in the plants, including many of the colorful pigments I wrote about in my earlier book, *What Color Is Your Diet?* However, when these fats are added to bleached white flour, starch, sugar, and artificial colors, their full inflammatory effect is present.

Atkins Confusion

The cholesterol-raising effects of saturated fats from meats and cheeses has been known for decades, but now the Atkins diet claims to lower cholesterol. In fact, this was the main message coming out of recent studies of the Atkins diet. What they don't tell you is that weight loss will usually result in lowering of cholesterol in susceptible groups of people. Many who have abdominal fat and a family history of diabetes will produce more triglycerides, due to the effects of high levels of insulin when they are overweight, than those with lower-body fat. The triglyceride is carried in a particle called a "very-low-density lipoprotein" that is 80 percent triglyceride and

20 percent cholesterol. When these people lose weight, their insulin levels go down and their triglyceride and cholesterol levels go down. Also for almost everyone: When you lower your total calorie intake and lose weight, calories trump the type of fat you are eating and cholesterol levels can fall. There are some people with high or low cholesterol who are resistant to diet changing their cholesterol levels, but in large groups of people, on average, weight loss causes a reduction in cholesterol levels. You see the differences among various types of fat only when the total calories in the diet are held constant. This explains why for decades saturated fat was associated with higher cholesterol when it was studied in people hospitalized and eating controlled diets, while it led to lower cholesterol levels in some people who were dieting on their own and cutting calories even while eating saturated fats from meats and cheeses.

Cancer and Polyunsaturated Fats

In animal studies, linoleic acid, which is found in corn oil and other vegetable fats, makes tumors grow and spread. It is likely this happens for two reasons. First, the linoleic acid can start a chain reaction of oxygen radical formation in cells, which can damage DNA, promoting cancer. Second, the linoleic acid is converted by cells into eicosanoids that can stimulate inflammation and contribute to causing cancer by damaging DNA. It is the ratio of omega-6 to omega-3 that determines these cell signals. Eating a lot of fruits and vegetables will balance these fatty acids against each other. However, a diet with lots of added polyunsaturated omega-6 fatty acids from hidden vegetable oils in processed foods is one factor among many that may be contributing to the increase in common forms of cancer seen when a population starts eating a diet rich in processed foods either because they move to the United States or we export our foods and lifestyle to them.

The Best Fat in Moderation

The news about dietary fat can seem pretty alarming, but there is a class of fats that is neutral for cholesterol and doesn't promote cancer: the monounsaturated fats found in olive oil and in avocados. You still need to consume these fats in moderation, because even the best of them have more than 120 calories per tablespoon. When I see people dipping bread in olive oil, I worry about their gaining weight. Just 3 tablespoons of olive oil contain close to 400 calories, which is a third of what some women need for the whole day.

Nonetheless, there are a number of studies in which the consumption of olive oil as part of the Mediterranean diet is associated with improved risks of heart disease and cancer. Avocado oil has the same healthy monounsaturated fats as olive oil. You would most likely get monounsaturated fats from avocados themselves rather than from their oil, which is only available for special cooking uses due to its expense. The number of calories per bite of avocado is equivalent to that found in chicken breast, and it can be included as a source of healthy fat in your diet without causing weight gain.

Was It a Big Fat Lie?

Were all the nutrition scientists lying to you all these years about fat making you fat? Absolutely not. Fats have been a major contribution to obesity in this country; they just weren't the whole story. We now know that the

The Science of Good Fats and Bad Fats

type of carbohydrate you eat is also important. Pasta, beans, rice, and potatoes can also make you fat, as mentioned in the section on glycemic index, glycemic load, and calories in Step 2. When you choose fats to add to your diet, calories still count. I try to be careful with my fat consumption by using olive oil pan spray for cooking or 1 or 2 tablespoons of oil for a large stir-fry of oriental vegetables, and I generally don't add olive oil to my salads. You can choose to eat these fats, but do try to burn all the fat you eat by exercising.

References

1.   Erkkila, A.T., Lehto, S., Pyorala, K., Uusitupa, M.I. "n-3 Fatty acids and 5-y risks of death and cardiovascular disease events in patients with coronary artery disease." *Am J Clin Nutr.* 2003 Jul;78(1):65–71.

2.   Food and Drug Administration, HHS. "Food labeling: trans fatty acids in nutrition labeling, nutrient content claims, and health claims. Final rule." *Federal Register.* 2003 Jul;11;68(133):41433–1506.

3.   Hu, F. "The Mediterranean diet and mortality—olive oil and beyond." *N Engl J Med.* 2003 Jun; 26;348(26):2595–96.

4.   Hu, F.B., Willett, W.C. "Optimal diets for prevention of coronary heart disease." *JAMA.* 2002 Nov; 27;288(20):2569–78.

5.   Simopoulos, A.P. "Omega-3 fatty acids in inflammation and autoimmune diseases." *J Am Coll Nutr.* 2002 Dec;21(6):495–505.

The Science of Cereals and Shakes

Many Americans have come to regard a bowl of cereal with milk and sliced banana and a glass of orange juice as the ultimate breakfast. Believe it or not, this breakfast contains 325 to 500 calories, with only 10 grams of protein:

    1 ounce bran cereal = 75 calories
    1 ounce raisin bran cereal = 190 calories
    Nonfat milk = 90 calories
    Low-fat milk = 120 calories
    Whole milk = 150 calories
    1 medium banana = 100 calories
    8 ounces orange juice = 160 calories

The low protein can leave you hungry in the midmorning. And what's worse, the calories listed above are for 1 ounce of cereal, and most people eat more than double the serving size. You may remember those tiny variety pack boxes. Those packages contain a 1-ounce serving. How does that compare to what you pour out of a cereal box? The high-protein principle (see the Appendix on the Science of Protein) and the need to control your calories at one or two meals a day on this program make the Empowering Shake your best choice. Not only will you get three times the protein, but also 5 grams of filling fiber with most fruits, and you will still end up eating under 300 calories for each shake. Science shows that this habit will help you keep your weight under control.

The bestselling cereals in America contain between 1 and 6 grams of protein (see the table on page 280). Granted, a full glass of milk would add another 10 grams, but what if you are just splashing your flakes with a little milk so that they are still crispy? You may only be getting one-sixth of the protein that the Empowering Shake gives you.

Can you still eat your favorite cereals as part of a high-protein breakfast? By adding 10 grams of protein from a protein powder (one with 5 grams of protein per tablespoon), you can make a higher-protein cereal without affecting the taste too much, especially if you are also adding fruit to the cereal. Among all the cereals, I believe that oatmeal has the best reputation for being a healthy cereal, even though some would argue for bran flakes, raisin bran, or a vitamin-fortified cereal. I base my assessment of consumer perceptions on the tremendous publicity given to the heart-healthy aspect of oatmeal marketing. However, I would fortify oatmeal with protein to make it a better occasional breakfast choice.

Eating oatmeal is a good habit when you consider the alternatives. In a restaurant, when you order the three-egg omelet with cheese, often you get a five-egg omelet. They don't tell you about the extra eggs because they want a satisfied customer eating big portions, and the extra eggs are cheaper than losing a customer. Someone else might order pancakes or Belgian waffles, which provide fat and carbohydrate with little protein. You could save up to 500 calories by ordering plain oatmeal instead of a heavy omelet or a big stack of pancakes. Sprinkle on a little brown sugar or a few raisins, top with a banana or other fruit, and add a splash of nonfat milk. You'll get that wonderful feeling that you're doing something healthy, since there is an approved health claim that oats reduce cholesterol.

It does matter which kind of oatmeal you choose. The kind you want is made from plain rolled oats, which are 100 percent whole grain and a good source of soluble fiber, the kind that lowers cholesterol and will keep you feeling full. Unfortunately, many people choose to eat instant oatmeal, which is usually loaded with sugar and artificial flavors and, in some cases, added fat. The little packets designated as a serving are so small that many people eat two. On the other hand, if you can survive the hunger and stick with a single serving, you may be able to lose weight using this as a sort of meal replacement. I wouldn't recommend doing this, since it leaves most people hungry by midmorning. I want you to lose weight without the usual hunger that accompanies other diets.

At home, you can make a bowl of protein-fortified oatmeal as an occasional alternative to your shake in the morning. However, it does contain 300 calories and 48 grams of carbohydrate, so moderation is key. Given the low-protein content of all oatmeals, I recommend also drinking a 12-ounce glass of milk with your oatmeal.

The Science of Cereals and Shakes

Protein-Fortified Oatmeal

SERVES 1

> 1 cup nonfat milk or plain soy milk
>
> Pinch of salt
>
> $^1/_3$ cup quick-cooking rolled oats (1 minute, not instant)
>
> 2 tablespoons vanilla-flavored soy protein powder
>
> Few dashes of cinnamon
>
> $^1/_2$ cup apple slices, raspberries, or blackberries, fresh or frozen, thawed, *or* $^1/_2$ sliced banana

1. Pour the milk or soy milk into a medium saucepan, add the salt, and place over medium-high heat. Bring the milk to a simmer (do not let it boil) and add the oats. Turn the heat to low and cook the oats, stirring, until thickened.

2. Stir in the protein powder, cinnamon, and the fruit, and stir 1 or 2 minutes, or until heated through. If the cereal is too thick, add a little extra nonfat milk or soy milk.

Nutrient Analysis per Serving (with nonfat milk and berries)
Calories: 300; Protein: 23 grams; Fat: 5 grams; Carbohydrate: 48 grams; Fiber: 10 grams

This recipe improves a good whole-fiber cereal by bringing the protein content up to 23 grams while taking advantage of the healthy aspects of oatmeal, including its great fiber. This is a much better choice than many of the best-selling cereals in America, which are listed in the chart in the next section.

The Bottom Line on Cereals Versus the Empowering Shake

If you are going to choose a cereal and add protein to it, it is still important to watch the amount of total carbohydrates and calories. Some cereals have 24 to 28 grams of carbohydrates, of which 11 or 12 grams are sugar. To make matters worse, some have only 1 or 2 grams of fiber, so you would need to add a fiber supplement or some fruit to feel full. Also, the number of calories varies greatly from 75 calories for some bran cereals to 190 calories for the popular Raisin Bran, which with two scoops of protein powder (40 calories) and a glass of milk (90 calories) adds up to 320 calories. With bran cereal (75 calories), you can cut the total calories for breakfast down to 215 calories, plus a half banana at 50 calories for a total 265 calories. As you can see, this gets complicated, and you will really throw things off if you eat a double serving of cereal, as so many people do.

My own solution over the last two years has been to get away from automatically eating cereal for breakfast. I do make my protein-fortified cereal occasionally, but more often, when I'm looking for a break from the Empowering Shake, I eat scrambled egg whites and sautéed vegetables or a cup of nonfat cottage cheese. However, the bottom line is still that to control your weight for a lifetime, for best results your everyday breakfast routine should include the Empowering Shake.

Cereal Nutrition Information

The information in the following table matches what you'll find on the nutrition labels for these cereals. Become a label reader and make good, informed choices if you're not having an Empowering Shake.

Food	Serving Size	Calories	Protein (grams)	Carbohydrate (grams)	Sugar (grams)	Fiber (grams)
Top Selling Cereals						
Frosted Flakes	¾ cup	120	1	28	12	1
Honey Nut Cheerios	1 cup	120	3	24	11	2
Frosted Mini-Wheats	18 mini-biscuits	150	4	36	9	4
Raisin Bran	1 cup	190	6	45	19	7
Lucky Charms	1 cup	120	2	25	13	1
Corn Flakes	1 cup	100	2	24	2	1
Cinnamon Toast Crunch	¾ cup	130	1	24	10	1
Rice Krispies	1 cup	100	2	23	2	0
High-Fiber and/or Higher Protein Cereals						
Nutlettes (Dixie Foods, 1-800-BEEFNOT)	½ cup	140	25	15	4	9
Kashi GOLEAN	¾ cup	120	8	28	7	10
All-Bran with Extra Fiber	¾ cup	75	5	30	0	18
Multi-Bran Chex	1 cup	200	4	49	12	7
All-Bran	½ cup	80	4	23	6	10
Oatmeal (Quick Rolled Oats)	⅓ cup	100	3	19	1	3
Plain Instant Oatmeal	1 packet	100	4	19	0	3
Shredded Wheat bite size	¾ cup	115	4	26	2	4
Kashi Good Friends	¾ cup	90	3	24	6	8
Kellogg Bran Buds	⅓ cup	70	2	24	8	13

The Science of Exercise and Building Muscle

Did you ever wonder how your muscles get the energy to work, or how best to build your muscles up? In this appendix I discuss how muscle works and how it relates to your diet and exercise regimen. There's a lot of information here, so if you find it overwhelming, come back to it later as you exercise more and learn more about your body. You can also use this information to see if things you are being told about exercise or muscle-building supplements make any sense.

Foods Become Fuel for Your Muscles

As you know, food contains protein, carbohydrate, and fat. The human body both breaks these elements into energy for chemical reactions and stores it through a complex interconnected network of chemical reactions or metabolic pathways. This carefully orchestrated network, which was established by your genes millions of years ago, is designed to provide the energy necessary for exercise. The network responds instantly to the state of your nutrition by monitoring your energy stores.

You store more than 160,000 calories of fat in your body, but only about 1,200 calories of carbohydrate as a starch (glycogen) in muscle and liver. Protein amino acids can be used to restore carbohydrates, but during exercise a well-nourished person uses fat or carbohydrate as the main fuel. Protein is normally spared from acting as a fuel, because the body keeps it in store for the emergency condition of starvation. If you eat no food, the length of time you will survive depends on how much lean body mass you have in your muscles and in organs such as the liver. Proteins play such an important role in maintaining your health that in cases of starvation or diseases such as cancer or AIDS that cause the body to use up its tissues for fuel, it is possible to predict the time of death as coinciding with the loss of 50 percent of a body's protein.

At low levels of prolonged exercise, most of our energy needs come from fat and lesser energy needs come from carbohydrate. Carbohydrate comes more into play with higher-intensity, short-duration exercise. Protein plays only a minor role at very high levels of energy utilization, but adequate protein intake is critical for maintaining your lean body mass to enable you to perform at your best. The exact degree to which either carbohydrate or fat acts as the primary or secondary source of energy, and the efficiency with which energy is used, depends on what you ate before you started exercising and the intensity and duration of the exercise. Less-trained individuals use carbohydrate earlier and will run out of energy earlier. The trained athlete's muscles are adapted to use fat efficiently and make the relatively scarce carbohydrate stores (1,200 calories versus 160,000 calories) last longer.

Inside the Muscle Cell: ATP and Creatine Phosphate

In order to understand how the muscle gets its energy, you need to know some basic facts about metabolism in the muscle cell. In all the cells of the body, including muscle cells, you extract energy from foods by converting the chemical energy stored within the chemical bonds holding carbohydrates, proteins, and fats together. The chemical energy stored in these bonds is released in a controlled manner for use by the body through metabolism. Metabolism is the collection of processes carried out by special proteins called "enzymes," which break down protein, carbohydrate, and fat into small chemicals. As this process continues, energy is stored in high-energy chemical bonds of foods, then removed and transferred in a highly controlled fashion to a special substance, ATP (adenosine triphosphate), so that the energy can ultimately be used to power living cells and to build complex substances like enzymes and fats for use in the cell. The adenosine in this chemical compound is the same one found in genetic material, but in ATP its main function is to serve as an anchor between two and three phosphate atoms. If there are two phosphates, the chemical compound is called "ADP" (adenosine diphosphate). For many of the energy-requiring processes in the body, such as making fats from fatty acids or proteins from amino acids, the energy from the third phosphate is released by converting ATP to ADP. This chemical energy is then available for the body processes that require energy and it is provided in a controlled way at the site where the energy-requiring reaction occurs so that there is minimal wasted energy or heat generated. In cells the ratio of ATP to ADP is an indication of the energy state of the cell, much as you would test the charge left in an alkaline battery in your flashlight. As ADP accumulates from use in energy-requiring reactions, the energy state of the cell would run down

The Science of Exercise and Building Muscle

just as a flashlight would dim with a run-down battery. Many energy-producing reactions in the body monitor the ATP-to-ADP ratio and regulate whether energy is being produced to restore the ATP used up by different processes. As ADP accumulates in the muscle, an enzyme is activated that breaks down phosphocreatine (PCr) in order to restore ATP levels (PCr + ADP $\longrightarrow$ ATP + Cr). The creatine released from this reaction is converted to creatinine and excreted in the urine. Phosphocreatine has this specialized function in muscle to enable muscle to restore ATP levels more quickly than is possible in other cells.

The stores of PCr in muscle are extremely limited and could only support muscle ATP levels for about 10 seconds if there were no other sources of ATP. Since ATP is provided from other sources, PCr ends up serving as a major energy source in only the first minute of strenuous exercise. PCr has the major advantage of being localized in the muscle, so that it can rapidly restore and maintain ATP levels during fast, intense exercises, such as sprinting, jumping, lifting, and throwing.

Aerobic and Anaerobic Metabolism

The body's chemical reactions that make ATP from food are classified as anaerobic (without oxygen) or aerobic (with oxygen). Aerobic metabolism is the most efficient means of extracting energy from food and uses oxygen within specialized structures called "mitochondria" to make 42 ATP molecules from a 6-carbon glucose molecule. In anaerobic metabolism, glucose is broken down without using oxygen. This is a simple but inefficient pathway that can only extract about 6 ATP molecules from breaking glucose down to lactate. While anaerobic metabolism can occur under very adverse conditions when oxygen is not available, such as in fatigued muscle, it's a second choice in humans (although it's the only alternative for primitive bacteria, which lack the machinery for aerobic metabolism).

At low to moderate levels of exercise, the body uses primarily aerobic metabolism, and only switches to anaerobic metabolism as it becomes exhausted or is faced with sudden huge muscle loads, as in competitive weight lifting. By using oxygen under most exercise conditions, the efficiency of the energy production from food-derived fuels in the cell is very much increased by comparison to what it would be with anaerobic metabolism.

In aerobic metabolism all the same steps used in anaerobic metabolism are carried out first but with one major difference—a key chemical produced from glucose called "pyruvate" is not converted into lactic acid, as it would be in anaerobic metabolism. Instead, pyruvate enters a biochemical pathway, the Krebs Cycle (named after the Nobel Prize winner Dr. Hans Krebs). The Krebs Cycle uses multiple chemicals and oxygen to amplify the energy as pyruvate is completely broken down to carbon dioxide and water. In the process, an additional 36 ATP molecules are produced, adding on to the 6 produced in the first part of the reaction for a total of 42 ATP molecules from one 6-carbon glucose molecule.

You can see how the mitochondria get their reputation as the energy factories of our cells, and muscle cells are particularly rich in mitochondria to provide the ATP needed for exercise. The mitochondria have their own cell walls and their own DNA. It is thought that they were originally some type of bacterial life form that was adopted by more complex cells to carry out the important function of producing energy from food and oxygen and releasing water and carbon dioxide. The reactions in the mitochondria are called "oxidative phosphorylation" and result in a maximum extraction of energy from each molecule of glucose.

If there is plenty of oxygen available and the exercise is of low to moderate intensity, then the pyruvate from glucose is converted to carbon dioxide and water in the mitochondria. Approximately 42 ATP equivalents can be produced from a single glucose molecule, compared to only 6 ATP with anaerobic metabolism. Aerobic metabolism supplies energy more slowly than anaerobic metabolism, but can be sustained for long periods of time—up to 5 hours. The major advantage of the less efficient anaerobic pathway is that it provides ATP in muscle more rapidly by using local muscle glycogen. Other than PCr, it is the fastest way to resupply ATP levels in the muscle. That is why anaerobic glucose metabolism is used by muscle cells in competitive weight lifting, in which a lot of energy is needed rapidly.

Anaerobic breakdown of glucose supplies most of the energy for intense short-term exercise, ranging from 30 seconds to 2 minutes. The disadvantage of anaerobic metabolism is that it cannot be sustained for long periods, since the accumulation of lactic acid in muscle decreases the pH and inactivates key enzymes in the glycolysis pathway, leading to fatigue. The lactic acid released from muscle can be taken up by the liver and converted to glucose again (the Cori Cycle), or it can be used as a fuel directly by the heart or by less active skeletal muscles, away from the actively contracting muscle.

Muscle Glycogen Stores and Exercise

Muscle glycogen is the preferred carbohydrate fuel for events lasting less than 2 hours for both aerobic and anaerobic metabolism. Depletion of muscle glycogen causes fatigue and is associated with a build-up of muscle lactate. Lactate production increases continuously, but physiologists have defined a point at which breathing changes as a result of acid-base imbalance, called the "anaerobic threshold." Both the nutrition and conditioning of the athlete will determine how much work can be performed in a specific exercise before fatigue sets in.

This can be measured directly or indirectly. An indirect measurement uses an exercise treadmill or stairway and takes the subject's pulse according to standard protocols. The more conditioned athlete can produce the same amount of work at a lower pulse rate. This indirect determination assumes that pulse rate is proportional to oxygen consumption. On the other hand, oxygen consumption can be measured directly during exercise. A motorized treadmill is usually used to increase the intensity of exercise as oxygen intake is measured until fatigue occurs. The maximal amount of oxygen consumed just before exhaustion is called the "VO_2max"—the most oxygen your body is capable of consuming.

Exercise intensity can be expressed as a percentage of VO_2max. Each individual has a personal VO_2max, which depends on their level of conditioning and how much lean body mass they have. A trained athlete with large muscles will have a much higher VO_2max than a sedentary worker who is not conditioned. Low-intensity exercises, such as fast walking, use 30 to 50 percent of VO_2max. Jogging can demand 50 to 80 percent of VO_2max, depending on the intensity, and sprints can require from 85 to 150 percent of VO_2max (with the added 50 percent coming from short-term anaerobic energy production). That is why the unconditioned person gets winded at a lower level of external work than the conditioned athlete.

It is possible to build up glycogen stores prior to exercise to improve performance. With exercises lasting for more than 20 to 30 minutes, blood glucose becomes important as a fuel to spare muscle glycogen breakdown. Both aerobic and endurance training lead to increases in glycogen stores, triglycerides, oxidative enzymes, and increased number and size of mitochondria.

How Muscle Adapts to Exercise

As you become conditioned to higher and higher levels of exercise, your muscle cells get bigger and develop the chemical machinery to carry out more energy production. Training increases both the enzymes that carry out the chemical reactions in the Krebs Cycle's oxidation of glucose and the lipoprotein lipase enzyme needed to convert triglycerides to fatty acids. This effect is specific to the muscle and muscle fiber type being used for the exercise.

Muscle fiber types are classified according to three characteristics: (1) the speed with which they can contract (fast or slow); (2) their content of glycogen and the enzymes necessary to produce energy through anaerobic metabolism; and (3) their content of mitochondria with oxidative enzymes for carrying out aerobic metabolism.

Slow-twitch muscle fibers are found in large muscles that maintain posture and stay contracted for long periods of time. They are red in color because they contain high concentrations of an oxygen-carrying protein called "myoglobin." They contain the chemical machinery to carry out aerobic metabolism slowly, which allows them to hold their position for long periods of time. Fast-twitch muscle fibers can contain a lot of glycogen for anaerobic metabolism, making them white (these are called type IIb fast-twitch fibers in the scientific literature). Another type of fast-twitch fiber (type IIa) has a combination of high speed with anaerobic metabolism necessary to break down glycogen for short energy bursts and aerobic capacity and oxidative enzymes in mitochondria for sustained activity.

Research has shown that with training it is possible to convert type IIb fibers into type IIa fast-twitch fibers, and that for a given activity the more type IIa fast-twitch fibers, the less fatigue will occur with prolonged exercise of that muscle group. In prolonged exercise at 60 to 75 percent of

VO$_2$max, type I fibers (red, slow-twitch) and type IIa (red, fast-twitch) are recruited during the early stages of exercise, but as the intensity increases, type IIb fibers (white, fast-twitch) must be recruited to maintain the same intensity. Then fatigue sets in when the type IIb fibers begin to release lactic acid—the product of anaerobic metabolism of the stored glycogen. This is what long-distance runners call "hitting the wall," as the lactic acid causes pain and fatigue in the muscles. As the glycogen levels drop in the red muscle fibers, they will rely more on your stores of fat. Since fat is less efficient than carbohydrate, the intensity of exercise will decrease, and your pace will slow.

Fat Fuels Early and Sustained Exercise

At the other end of the spectrum, during mild exercise such as a brisk walk, muscles burn fat for fuel because the supply of ATP provided from fat is adequate to maintain intensity. Fatty acids are readily available from stored fat, and the rate of breakdown of stored fat is three times the rate of fatty acid release at rest, so that fatty acids can be supplied at an increased rate rapidly during low levels of exercise. So, while fat is not very useful for short-term, intense exercise, it is a great advantage for prolonged exercise, especially at a low or moderate level of intensity.

The advantage of fat as a fuel is that it provides extensive stores of calories in a easily portable form. Since fat is not hydrated, it weighs much less per unit calorie than protein or carbohydrate (9 cal/gm of fat versus 4 cal/gm of carbohydrate or protein). When you compare the number of ATP produced per carbon atom, fat is also more efficient. A 6-carbon glucose molecule produces 36 to 38 ATP on average, providing a ratio of 6 ATP/carbon, while an 18-carbon fatty acid produces 147 ATP, providing a ratio of 8.2

The Science of Exercise and Building Muscle

ATP/carbon. However, carbohydrate is more efficient than fat when the amount of ATP produced per unit of oxygen consumed is considered. Six oxygen molecules are required to metabolize 6-carbon glucose, producing 36 ATP (ratio = 6 ATP/oxygen molecule), while 26 oxygen molecules are required to produce 147 ATP from an 18-carbon fatty acid (5.7 ATP/oxygen molecule). Therefore, for a performance athlete it is important to maintain the efficiency edge provided by carbohydrate as long as glycogen is available in the muscles. Under usual exercise conditions, protein provides only about 6 percent of energy needs. With high-intensity endurance exercise, the production of glucose from amino acids can be significant—up to about 10 or 15 percent of total energy needs. The only food that provides energy for short-term fast-paced exercise is carbohydrate, while slow, steady aerobic exercise uses all three primary fuels (but primarily fat and carbohydrate).

How Much Exercise Is Enough?

The practical application of the preceding information falls into two categories: first, the prescription of adequate amounts of exercise to optimize performance and second, what is known about building muscle most effectively.

The Exercise Prescription

The components of fitness are flexibility, strength, endurance, and cardiovascular fitness or endurance.

- Flexibility is the ability to bend without injury, which is dependent on the elasticity of muscles, tendons, ligaments, and joints. Stretching for at least 10 seconds with gradual tension will improve flexibility.

- Strength is the ability to work against resistance. Strength of particular muscle groups can be increased by careful heavy resistance training.

- Endurance is the ability to sustain effort over a period of time. High-repetition exercises such as push-ups, pull-ups, and sit-ups increase endurance.

- Cardiovascular fitness or endurance is the ability of the heart, lungs, and blood vessels to sustain effort over a period of time.

A basic exercise prescription involves a stretching session and a 10-minute low-intensity warm-up to increase blood flow and minimize risk of injury. That is followed by exercises to increase muscular strength, endurance, and flexibility. These exercises should be performed at an intensity adequate to increase the heart rate into a training zone, which is 60 to 90 percent of maximum age-adjusted heart rate (MHR = 220 minus your age in years) (see Step 6, page 169). I usually start individuals at 50 to 60 percent of MHR, and then keep them in that training zone. For weight loss, prolonged sessions at 70 percent of MHR are effective at burning fat, while increased levels of exercise induce the muscles being used to grow. A 10-minute cool-down is important to minimize cramping and muscle injury at the end of each session.

A gradual incremental exercise program emphasizing cardiovascular fitness is the basis of all exercise programs. Vigorous exercise involves minimal risks for healthy individuals, but can be risky for couch potatoes. These people should check with their physician first, as should all those over thirty-five or with medical conditions such as arthritis, hypertension, shortness of breath, diabetes, or a family history of heart disease. In gen-

The Science of Exercise and Building Muscle

eral, it is a good idea to check with your doctor before starting an exercise program even if you are just healthy and overweight.

How Many Calories Are Burned?

Exercise output can be quantified as METs, which are a ratio of the energy being burned to that burned at rest. An individual at rest burns about 1 cal/per kg/per hour (depending on lean body mass content), and this rate equals one MET. Therefore, a 50-kilogram (110-pound) woman would expend about 10 METs if she was in a heavy aerobics exercise class burning 500 cal/hour.

$$\frac{500 \text{ calories/hour}}{1 \text{ cal/kg times } 50 \text{ kg}} = 10 \text{ METs}$$

TYPICAL MET LEVELS (FOR COMPARISON ONLY, SINCE THEY DIFFER BY INDIVIDUAL)

For a 130-pound woman:	Activity	MET level	Calories/Hour
	Writing	1.7	103
	Walking	4	260
	Basketball	10	473
	Bicycling	3	178
	Eating	1.4	81
	Jogging	7	414
	Weight lifting	9	532

The main uses of METs are in comparing exercises performed by individuals in different programs and to test fitness on standard treadmill tests. In any individual, the resting energy expenditure will depend on muscle mass, and the amount of energy expended will depend on level of training. So this is only an approximate measure of fitness or the calories expended in any activity.

Building Muscle: Strength-Training Basics

In the last fifteen years, better strength training programs have been developed as scientists learned more about how to maximize muscle building over the long term. Studies have shown that over the first twelve weeks, doing three sets of 8 to 10 repetitions of weight-lifting exercises at 60 to 80 percent of the maximum weight you can lift has as good a result as more scientific programs, such as periodized resistance training, in which workouts are created that vary in intensity, repetition, and rest and recovery periods. The difference shows up when you look at results over six months to a year.

Individualization is an important principle of training, just as it's important to individualize metabolism and protein requirements on the L.A. Shape Diet. Baseline testing of your muscle strength is needed to determine which muscle groups need strengthening. The next step is to develop realistic, specific, and individual goals. Sound familiar? So, your expectations for improvement can be framed in terms of time and ultimate muscle bulk or strength desired.

Specific movements and tasks train groups of muscles involved in those complex movements. The type of muscle fiber recruited to the movement also depends on how much external weight is being lifted. Endurance exercises at low weights and high repetitions recruit the type 1 slow-twitch fibers while heavier exercises recruit the type 2 fast-twitch fibers as well.

There are three different types of muscle contractions: isometric, isotonic, and eccentric. An isometric contraction is basically a contraction that holds the muscle in the same position with no motion of the joint. However, the muscles still contract as when you tighten your abdomen while standing without doing a sit-up or crunch. You tighten the muscle and hold for 10 seconds. Then you relax. The muscle has worked but has not resulted in movement. A simple biceps arm curl is an isotonic exercise that produces an isotonic contraction of the biceps muscle. Joint motion occurs at the elbow as the muscle shortens with the isotonic muscle contraction. An eccentric contraction is a controlled lengthening action of the muscle. Eccentric contractions occur to decelerate the body and absorb shock. The quadriceps muscle (the muscle in front of the top of the thigh) undergoes an eccentric contraction when it lands on the ground after jumping off a 12-inch box.

Pylometric exercises (jumping, hopping, catching weighted balls) require eccentric contractions of some muscles groups to complete a specific activity by acting against the dominant movement of the muscle action. You should not experience pain in your workouts, but you need to stimulate your muscles to grow by increasing the demands you make on them at every session. The muscle fibers are stretched on the down cycle of a biceps curl. So, the sequence of timing should be 2 seconds on the upswing and a slower controlled 4 seconds on the downswing. For other exercises, you need to decide which is the eccentric movement for the muscle you are trying to train. On the last few repetitions, you should feel a slight burning on the eccentric move.

The term for this is "progressive overload," which simply means that if you were comfortable doing 10 repetitions of an exercise, now go to 11. The way to measure this scientifically is to use the 1-repetition maximum, or 1RM. The external weights at which you can do 5 repetitions is called the 5RM; the weight at 10 repetitions, 10RM; and so forth. The RM system has been used for more than fifty years to describe resistance-exercise intensities. In a famous paper, Thomas L. DeLorme and A. L. Watkins documented the importance of progressive resistance exercise to build the quadriceps muscles for the purpose of rehabilitating military personnel with knee injuries.

An RM training zone of 8 to 10RM is the general level used by most trainers, but in order to continue to improve, variation is needed, and that is where periodized training comes in. The intensities for different types of training days are listed below:

Very Heavy: Develop maximal 1RM strength by doing three to five sets of 2 to 4 repetitions and resting 4 minutes or more between sets.

Moderate: Develop strength and increase muscle size and some endurance by doing three sets of 8 to 10 repetitions with 2 or 3 minutes rest between sets.

Power Training: Develop maximal mechanical power in a multiple-joint exercise, such as throwing a medicine ball, by doing three to six sets of 3 repetitions at 30 to 50 percent of the 1RM with 3 or 4 minutes rest between sets.

Very Light: Develop local muscle endurance by doing two sets of 15 to 17 repetitions with less than 1 minute of rest between sets.

High Lactic Acid: Develop tolerance of lactic acid accumulation in muscles, which normally causes fatigue and soreness, by doing three sets of 8 to 10 repetitions with only 1 or 2 minutes rest between sets.

Periodized training on a four-day-per-week workout schedule could consist of the following:

Monday: Vary the training from heavy (3 to 5RM) to moderate (8 to 10RM) to light (12 to 15 RM) on successive days.

Tuesday: Train with moderate loads of 8 to 10 repetitions.

Thursday: Vary the training from heavy (3 to 5RM) to moderate (8 to 10RM) to light (12 *to 15 RM) on successive days.*

Friday: Train with moderate loads of 8 to 10 repetitions.

If more repetitions than the target can be achieved, the resistance can be increased for the next session. When this type of regimen was tested in college-age women against simply working out three alternate days per week at 8 to 10 repetitions, after six months there was a clear advantage for this periodized method. At twelve weeks, both methods worked, so really this is an advanced course for those who want to maximize their L.A. Shape.

For most exercisers, varying the routine by employing different strategies on different days reduces boredom and tends to keep them involved in the training program. This model has been proven to be superior to using the same repetition maximum in every workout.

Finally, it's important to note that you will get the maximum effects and the least likelihood of injury if your workouts are supervised to be sure you are doing each exercise correctly. The American College of Sports Medicine (ACSM) certifies health and fitness instructors, and this certification should be a minimum requirement for the trainer you choose. I would also get personal recommendations, as you would with any professional you consult.

References

1. DeLorme, T. "Restoration of muscle power by heavy resistance exercises." *J. Bone and Joint Surgery.* 1945;26:645–67.

    The classic paper demonstrating muscle building through strength training.

2.	Marx, J.O., Ratamess, N.A., Nindl, B.C., et al. "Low-volume circuit versus high-volume periodized resistance training in women." *Med Sci Sports Exerc.* 2001;33:635–43.

	This paper proves that periodized training works better after six months.

3.	Selye, H.A. "Syndrome produced by various noxious agents." *Nature.* 1936;138:32.

	The theory of stress and adaptation that forms the basis for all muscle building as the muscle adapts to an external stress in training that is constantly changed.

4.	Sherman, W., Costill, D., Fink W., et al. "Effect of exercise-diet manipulation on muscle glycogen and its subsequent utilization during performance." *Int J Sports Med.* 1981; 2:114.

	This paper explains the use of carbohydrate in exercise.

The following three papers use exercise testing to investigate energy use in muscles and carbohydrate loading as a maneuver to increase performance.

Coggan, A.R., Coyle, E.F. "Carbohydrate ingestion during prolonged exercise: effects on metabolism and performance." *Exerc Sports Sci Rev.* 1991;19:1–40.

Ivy, J., Katz, A.L., Cutler, C.L., et al. "Muscle glycogen synthesis after exercise: effect of time of carbohydrate ingestion." *J Appl Physiol.* 1988; 64:1480–85.

Murray, R., Paul, G.L., Siefert, J.G., et al. "Responses to varying rates of carbohydrate ingestion after exercise." *Med Sci Sports Exerc.* 1991;23: 713–18.

The Science of Exercise and Building Muscle

The Science of Vitamins and Minerals

There is still controversy about vitamins in newspapers and medical journals in this country, which reflects the poor state of nutrition education in our medical schools. Studies in which vitamins are compared to drugs are publicized as showing that vitamins have no benefit, and many physicians and other health-care providers are not familiar with the significant body of scientific studies supporting the use of vitamins and minerals.

The majority of Americans do not meet through their diets the recommended daily allowance (RDA) of many of the vitamins and minerals that are critical to health promotion and disease prevention. Vitamin supplementation has been shown to prevent neural tube defects and improve immune function, and other studies suggest that generous intake of vitamins and minerals may reduce the risk of coronary heart disease, cancer, and osteoporosis. I believe science will ultimately provide the final proof that optimal intakes of vitamins and minerals are important goals in efforts at disease prevention and health promotion. The available data are sufficiently strong for me to recommend confidently that you take vitamin and mineral supplements, and in this appendix I describe some of the scientific evidence that vitamins and minerals help your health.

There are three scientific arguments supporting the use of vitamins and mineral supplements. First, they can help bring consumption of vitamins and minerals up to recommended levels. Second, there may be benefits of vitamins and minerals for maintaining optimal health and preventing disease at levels above the recommended intakes. Finally, adequate micronutrient intake can be beneficial in reducing the risk of birth defects and may help reduce the risk of some chronic diseases.

These concepts are grounded in evidence provided by a large number of laboratory studies and population studies, and a small number of clinical trials. Additional research looking at dosing levels, targeted populations, and long-term effects is now under way.

Pregnancy and Birth Defects

One out of every thirty babies born in the United States has a serious birth defect. Each year, some 3,000 pregnancies are affected by a neural tube defect (NTD), such as spina bifida (an opening in the spinal cord that does not close) or anencephaly (a baby born without a brain).

Since 1980, more than a dozen studies have examined the role of folic acid in reducing the incidence of neural tube defects. Perhaps the most important, the 1991 United Kingdom Medical Research Council randomized clinical trial, found that folic acid use could reduce the relative risk of NTD by more than 70 percent (MRC Vitamin Study Research Group). The United States Public Health Service drew on these data to issue recommendations on folic acid the following year. They said that women capable of becoming pregnant should take 400 micrograms (or millionths of a gram) of folic acid daily, which is the amount contained in a daily multivitamin. The Food and Drug Administration followed this advisory with orders requiring all products made with "enriched" grain to contain additional folic acid and approved the use of health claims for products that contain significant amounts of the vitamin. The Centers for Disease Control and Prevention (CDC) suggest that the consumption of supplemental folic acid could significantly reduce that number even beyond what has been achieved to date with the fortification of "enriched" grain products—to the extent that about 80 percent of these birth defects could be prevented.

Educational programs soon emerged, targeting women of childbearing years, health-care professionals, women's groups, and policy makers. Studies conducted in China, Canada, and the United States have shown that fortification programs have dramatically lowered the prevalence of NTD. More and more women of childbearing age have become familiar with the need for folic acid; the percentage of women between eighteen and forty-five who learned about folic acid grew by more than 50 percent between 1995 and 2000. However, only 10 percent knew the correct dose and only one-third actually consumed the vitamin daily. Thus, although at least part of the folic acid message is reaching targeted women, not all are benefiting from that information.

Immune Function

Diet and nutritional status are two of the key factors affecting the body's immune response. Recent studies show that multivitamin use, in concert with a good diet, is a cost-effective tool to enhance immunity, reduce the incidence of infection, and improve overall quality of life. Immune status is relatively easy to test because unlike in cardiovascular disease or cancer, established and accepted measures of immune function are available. In randomized clinical trials conducted by Dr. Ranjit Chandra in Newfoundland, Canada, micronutrients have been shown to enhance the response of lymphocytes and natural killer cells, to increase production of the cytokine, interleukin-2, and to reduce the duration of infection and the time spent on antibiotics. These studies demonstrate that inadequate micronutrient intakes are associated with poorer immune responses and an increased incidence of infection, and that consumption of a multivitamin can help eliminate this deficit.

Cardiovascular Disease

Elevated levels of homocysteine are a major risk factor for coronary disease and ischemic stroke. Indeed, people with the highest homocysteine levels have a nearly twofold increase in the risk of coronary heart disease (CHD), compared to those with normal levels. This risk is comparable to that associated with smoking or high cholesterol. Folate is essential to homocysteine metabolism, and a number of studies have established the link between folate intake and CHD. Contributions to lowering homocysteine levels are also made, though to a lesser degree, by vitamins B_6 and B_{12}. Low-serum folate levels were associated with an increased risk of fatal CHD in studies from Canada (Morrison) and Europe (Robinson), while in the United States, higher intake of folate and vitamin B_6 reduced that risk (Rimm). Homocysteine-lowering therapy with folate and B complex was also found to decrease the incidence of death, nonfatal heart attacks, and other adverse events following coronary angioplasty (Schnyder). This finding was confirmed in a large case-control study from Sweden, which showed that use of a multivitamin supplement reduced the risk of a myocardial infarction by 21 percent in men and 34 percent in women, suggesting that consumption of folate and B complex may aid in the primary prevention of heart attacks (Holmquist). Additional studies are now in progress to further clarify the relationship between these vitamins and coronary disease.

Vitamins C and E are essential well-established antioxidants, and researchers have investigated whether these micronutrients have a role to play in heart disease prevention. To date, some studies have found a mild effect for higher-dose vitamin C users (Osganian), while others have failed to establish a relationship (Kushi). Similarly, the Nurses' Health Study found that women taking modest amounts of vitamin E had a 44 percent reduction in the incidence of heart disease (Stampfer) and that higher doses (400–800 IU) reduced the rate of second heart attacks in heart patients (Stephens). However, other well-controlled trials found no effect (Rapola; Yusuf).

Since these studies were done in individuals who already had heart disease, it is difficult to account for the many different factors that may have caused their heart disease and made them different from one another. Therefore, when these people were assigned by chance to get the placebo or vitamin supplements, the results may have been related more to the individual profiles of those assigned to the two arms of the study than to whether the vitamins were having an effect. Researchers assumed that such differences are overcome by large numbers, but this may not be true in the case of a complex disease such as heart disease, with so many different factors involved. While it would be of great interest to conduct a prevention study in otherwise healthy individuals, such a study would require huge numbers and be prohibitively expensive.

Cancer

Folate deficiency may contribute to the development of cancer by interfering with normal gene processes. Thus, there has been much recent interest in the effects of folate supplementation on cancer prevention. Both the Nurses Health Study and the Health Prodessional Follow-up Study found that long-term (15 years in the former, 10 in the latter) folate consumption signficantly reduced the risk of colorecttal cancer. Moderate drinkers who were folate deficient saw an even greater reduction (Giovannucci, Annals Int Med, 1998; Giovannucci, 1995). Among women who use alchol and have low blood folate levels, supplementation helped lower the elevated risk of breast cancer associated with drinking (Zhang). Ongoing trials are continuing to explore the effects of folate supplementation, especially in users of alcohol, where the interaction appears to be very strong.

Vitamin E has been investigated in connection with a number of major cancers, including breast, lung, colon, and prostate. Only in the latter cancer does vitamin E appear to have a significant effect across several studies. In the ATBC (Alpha-Tocopherol Beta-Carotene) trial, researchers found that 400 milligrams of vitamin E reduced the incidence of, as well as mortality from, prostate cancer in male smokers (Albanes). This association has since been confirmed, both in nonsmokers and smokers. On the strength of this evidence, the National Cancer Institute is conducting a primary prevention trial of selenium and vitamin E versus a placebo for prostate cancer prevention in 25,000 normal men called the SELECT trial.

An editorial in the *New York Times* suggested that no cancer patients should take vitamin C or vitamin E, but it was based on a misinterpretation of two basic findings. The first is that vitamin C is concentrated by cancer cells, which they assumed meant that the cancer cell used this vitamin C to stimulate tumor cell growth. Dr. David Golde of Sloan-Kettering Cancer

Center in New York discovered that vitamin C was taken up by the glucose transport proteins in tumor cells. Before the tumor cell can take up vitamin C through the glucose transport system, it must be oxidized to a form called "dehydroascorbate." This form of vitamin C is taken up and then is trapped in the cell, where it is converted back to vitamin C inside the cell by reducing enzymes. But the concentrations required to do this do not occur in humans who take vitamin C orally; to reach these concentrations, vitamin C has to be given intravenously. This would never happen in someone taking vitamin supplements. The experiments that resulted in the caution on vitamin E were performed in animals that were made vitamin E deficient and compared to normal vitamin E status animals. Because it is not possible to make humans deficient in vitamin E, this study also has no relevance to supplements of vitamin E in humans with cancer.

The consumption of various carotenoids, such as lycopene, lutein, and beta-carotene, may reduce the risk of lung cancer by one-third, but pure beta-carotene at high doses of 30 milligrams may elevate it, particularly in smokers. Calcium supplementation, too, may protect against osteoporosis and the development and recurrence of colon polyps, which are a precancerous change in the colon (Baron; Bonithon-Kopp), but some data suggest that in extremely high doses (greater than 1,500 milligrams per day total), calcium may increase the risk of prostate cancer (Chan; Giovannucci, *Cancer Research*, 1998). Data in the latter study suggested that taking vitamin D with calcium may reduce any negative effects while maintaining the colon cancer protection. Also, no man should get less than the recommended dietary allowance, which is 1,000 milligrams per day of calcium. Cancer is a collection of heterogeneous conditions with complex causes and histories, and there is much more research that needs to be done on the use of vitamins and minerals for cancer prevention.

Obesity and Diabetes

While most of the population fails to consume adequate levels of micronutrients, the problem is particularly severe for the obese. There is evidence that overweight men and women with high cholesterol levels who are on diets do not achieve the recommended daily allowance of most essential vitamins and minerals, due to lower micronutrient intake, lack of adherence, and overrestriction of foods (Gryzbek). This nutritional deficiency clearly compromises their health status. Research conducted on people with type II diabetes has shown that those taking a multivitamin supplement had a lower incidence of infections and infection-related absenteeism than did those receiving placebo (Barringer). While a relatively small study, the magnitude of the differences in infection incidence noted over one year in diabetic patients was remarkable. Those who took a placebo had a 93 percent incidence over one year of infectious episodes, while those taking a multivitamin had an incidence of only 17 percent. These findings deserve further research in larger populations, as the implications are significant. In a study of people at risk for diabetes, investigators reported that males who took beta-carotene supplements improved their glucose metabolism, as did women who consumed vitamin E (Ylonen). While dieting has important implications for nutritional intake in all populations, it may play an even more essential role in those who are overweight and those with either metabolic syndrome or adult-onset diabetes mellitus.

Safety of Vitamins

The consumption of vitamin A above 25,000 IU per day (daily value = 5,000 IU) can clearly cause skeletal birth defects—and this amount is only five times the RDA. Pregnant women should not consume more than

2,500 IU of vitamin A per day to avoid any possibility of problems. A few recent studies suggest that long-term consumption in excess of 5,000 IU per day of vitamin A may also be associated with decreased bone mineral density and an increased risk of osteoporosis (Promislow). On the other hand, insufficient intake also may accelerate the loss of bone mineral density. Thus, there is a narrow window of optimal vitamin A intake in adults. I recommend that you use a multivitamin that contains about 2,500 IU of preformed vitamin A, or 5,000 IU of vitamin A, of which at least 50 percent comes from beta-carotene.

As noted previously, high calcium intakes (above 1,500 milligrams per day) have been associated with an increased risk of prostate cancer (Giovannucci, *Cancer Research*, 1998). An antioxidant supplement combining vitamins C and E, selenium, and beta-carotene was found to reduce the protective effects of a lipid-lowering agent and niacin in 160 patients with heart disease and low HDL cholesterol levels (Brown), although a larger trial of 20,000 patients, using a supplement of vitamin C, vitamin E, and beta-carotene, reported that the antioxidant combination did not inhibit the protective effects of the lipid-lowering drug (Heart Protection Study Collaborative Group).

Conclusion

I recommend vitamins to my patients and family, and I take vitamins myself. The scientific evidence supporting the intake of vitamins and minerals is growing and is based on sound science.

References

1. Albanes, D., Heinonen, O.P., Huttunen, J.K., Taylor, P.R., Virtamo, J., Edwards, B.K., Haapakoski, J., Rautalahti, M., Hartman, A.M., Palmgren, J., et al. "Effects of alpha-tocopherol and beta-carotene supplements on cancer incidence in the Alpha-Tocopherol Beta-Carotene Cancer Prevention Study." *Am J Clin Nutr.* 1995;62 (Suppl 6):1427S–1430S.

2. Baron, J.A., Beach, M., Mandel, J.S, et al. "Calcium supplements for the prevention of colorectal adenomas." *N Engl J Med.* 1999; 340:101–07.

3. Barringer, T.A., Kirk, J.K., Santaniello, A.C., Foley, K.L., Michielutte, R. "Effect of a multivitamin and mineral supplement on infection and quality of life. A randomized, double-blind, placebo-controlled trial." *Ann Intern Med.* 2003;138(5):365–71.

4. Bonithon-Kopp, C., Kronborg, O., Giacosa, A., Rath, U., Faivre, J. "Calcium and fibre supplementation in prevention of colorectal adenoma recurrence: a randomised intervention trial." European Cancer Prevention Organisation Study Group. *Lancet.* 2000;356(9238):1300–06.

5. Brown, B.G., Zhao, X.Q., Chait, A., Fisher, L.D., Cheung, M.C., Morse, J.S., Dowdy, A.A., Marino, E.K., Bolson, E.L., Alaupovic, P., Frohlich, J., Albers, J.J. "Simvastatin and niacin, antioxidant vitamins, or the combination for the prevention of coronary disease." *N Engl J Med.* 2001;Nov; 29; 345(22):1583–92.

6. Chan, J.M., Pietinen, P., Virtanen, M., Malila, N., Tangrea, J., Albanes, D., Virtamo, J. "Diet and prostate cancer risk in a cohort of

The Science of Vitamins and Minerals

smokers, with a specific focus on calcium and phosphorus (Finland)." *Cancer Causes Control.* 2000;Oct;11(9):859–67.

7. Chandra, R.K. "Effect of vitamin and trace-element supplementation on immune responses and infection in elderly subjects." *Lancet.* 1992;340:1124–27.

8. Giovannucci, E., Rimm, E.B., Wolk, A., Ascherio, A., Stampfer, M.J., Colditz, G.A., Willett, W.C. "Calcium and fructose intake in relation to risk of prostate cancer." *Cancer Res.* 1998;58(3):442–47.

9. Giovannucci, E., Stampfer, M.J., Colditz, G.A., Hunter, D.J., Fuchs, C., et al. "Multivitamin use, folate, and colon cancer in women in the Nurses' Health Study." *Ann. Intern Med.* 1998;129(7):517–24.

10. Graham, I.M., Daly, L.E., Refsum, H.M., Robinson, K., Brattstrom, L.E., et al. "Plasma homocysteine as a risk factor for vascular disease." The European Concerted Action Project. *JAMA.* 1997;277(22):1775–81.

11. Gryzbek, A., Klosiewicz-Latoszek, L., Targosz, U. "Changes in the intake of vitamins and minerals by men and women with hyperlipidemia and overweight during dietetic treatment." *Eur J Clin Nutr.* 2002;56:1162–68.

12. Heart Protection Study Collaborative Group. "MRC/BHF Heart Protection Study of antioxidant vitamin supplementation in 20,536 high-risk individuals: a randomised placebo-controlled trial." *Lancet.* 2002;360(9326):23–33.

13. Holmquist, C., Larsson, S., Wolk, A., deFaire, U. "Multivitamin supplements are inversely associated with risk of myocardial infarction

in men and women." Stockholm Heart Epidemiology Program (SHEEP). *J Nutr.* 2003;133:2650–54.

14. Kushi, L.H., Folsom, A.R., Prineas, R.J., Mink, P.J., Wu, Y., et al. "Dietary antioxidant vitamins and death from coronary heart disease in postmenopausal women." *N Engl J Med.* 1996;334(18):1156–62.

15. Michaud, D.S., Feskanich, D., Rimm, E.B., Colditz, G.A., Speizer, F.E., Willett, W.C., Giovannucci, E. "Intake of specific carotenoids and risk of lung cancer in 2 prospective US cohorts." *Am J Clin Nutr.* 2000;72(4):990–97.

16. Morrison, H.I., Schaubel, D., Desmeules, M., Wigle, D.T. "Serum folate and risk of fatal coronary heart disease." *JAMA.* 1996; 275(24):1893–96.

17. MRC Vitamin Study Research Group. "Prevention of neural tube defects: results of the Medical Research Council Vitamin Study." *Lancet.* 1991;338(8760):131–37.

18. Osganian, S.K., Stampfer, M.J., Rimm, E., Spiegelman, D., Hu, F.B., Manson, J.E., Willett, W.C. "Vitamin C and risk of coronary heart disease in women." *J Am Coll Cardiol.* 2003;42(2):246–52.

19. Persad, V.L., Van den Hof, M.C., Dube, J.M., Zimmer, P. "Incidence of open neural tube defects in Nova Scotia after folic acid fortification." *CMAJ.* 2002;167(3):241–45.

20. Promislow, J.H., Goodman-Gruen, D., Slymen, D.J., Barrett-Connor, E. "Retinol intake and bone mineral density in the elderly: the Rancho Bernardo Study." *J Bone Miner Res.* 2002;17(8):1349–58.

21. Rapola, J.M., Virtamo, J., Ripatti, S., Huttunen, J.K., Albanes, D., Taylor, P.R., Heinonen, O.P. "Randomised trial of alpha-tocopherol and beta-carotene supplements on incidence of major coronary events in men with previous myocardial infarction." *Lancet.* 1997;349(9067):1715–20.

22. Rimm, E.B., Willett, W.C., Hu, F.B., Sampson, L., Colditz, G.A., et al. "Folate and vitamin B$_6$ from diet and supplements in relation to risk of coronary heart disease among women." *JAMA.* 1998; 279(5):359–64.

23. Robinson, K., Arheart, K., Refsum, H., Brattstrom, L., Boers, G., et al. "Low circulating folate and vitamin B$_6$ concentrations: risk factors for stroke, peripheral vascular disease, and coronary artery disease." European COMAC Group. *Circulation.* 1998;97(5):437–43.

24. Schnyder, G., Roffi, M., Flammer, Y., Pin, R., Hess, O. "Effect of homocystein-lowering therapy with folic acid, vitamin B$_{12}$ and vitamin B$_6$ on clinical outcome after percutaneous coronary intervention." The Swiss Heart Study: A Randomized Controlled Trial. *JAMA.* 2002;288:973–79.

25. Stampfer, M., Hennekens, C., Manson, J., Colditz, G., Rosner, B., et al. "Vitamin E consumption and the risk of coronary artery disease in women." *N. Engl J Med.* 1993;328(20):1444–49.

26. Stephens, N.G., Parsons, A., Schofield, P.M., Kelly, F., Cheeseman, K., et al. "Randomised controlled trial of vitamin E in patients with coronary disease: Cambridge Heart Antioxidant Study (CHAOS)." *Lancet.* 1996;347(9004):781–86.

27. "Summary of notifiable diseases—United States, 2000." *MMWR Morb Mortal Wkly Rep.* 2002;Jun; 14:49(53):i–xxii, 1–100.

Appendix

28. Ylonen, K., Alfthan, G., Groop, L., Saloranta, C., Aro, A., Virtanen, S.M. "Dietary intakes and plasma concentrations of carotenoids and tocopherols in relation to glucose metabolism in subjects at high risk of type 2 diabetes: the Botnia Dietary Study." *Am J Clin Nutr.* 2003; 77(6):1434–41.

29. Yusuf, S., Dagenais, G., Pogue, J., Bosch, J., Sleight, P. "Vitamin E supplementation and cardiovascular events in high-risk patients." The Heart Outcomes Prevention Evaluation Study Investigators. *N Engl J Med.* 2000;342(3):154–60.

30. Zhang, S., Hunter, D.J., Hankinson, S.E., Giovannucci, E.L., Rosner, B.A., Colditz, G.A., Speizer, F.E., Willett, W.C. "A prospective study of folate intake and the risk of breast cancer." *JAMA.* 1999; 281(17):1632–37.

Worksheet and Daily Diary

How to Use Your Personal Diary

- If possible, have your body composition measured by bioelectrical impedance analysis.

- For each pound of lean body mass you have, you should eat an equivalent number of grams of protein per day, rounded to the nearest 25 grams (i.e., if you have 105 pounds of lean body mass, your goal would be 100 grams of protein per day, or 4 protein units; if you have 168 pounds of lean body mass, your goal would be 175 grams of protein).

- Your lean body mass will also determine your Resting Metabolic Rate (RMR), or the number of calories you burn per day at rest. If you are inactive, you probably don't burn many more calories than the RMR, so you would subtract 500 calories per day from your RMR to establish your daily target calorie level, which would allow you to lose about a pound per week.

If Your Target Weight Seems Too High

- If this target weight seems too high to you, then you have more muscle than the average person of your height. You should try to maintain the extra muscle by doing strength training as well as aerobic exercise.

If Your Target Weight Seems Too Low

- If this target weight seems too low, then you may have been inactive due to an injury or illness, or you may have eaten too little protein on previous crash diets. Since each pound of lean body mass burns about 14 calories/day, you should attempt to build up your muscle through weight lifting to increase the number of calories you are burning. For example, if you built 10 pounds of muscle over one year, your metabolism would increase by 140 calories per day.

- If you are unable to have your body composition measured, use the tables on pages 48 and 49 to estimate your lean body mass and protein requirements. Find the number of protein units that most closely matches your estimated lean body mass, and use the following chart to plan the calories and portions from each food group you need each day.

	Protein Units (25 grams each)	Fruits	Vegetables	Grains
Daily Target Calories	Number of Units	Number of Units	Number of Units	Number of Units
1,200	4	3	4	1
1,500	6	3	4	2
1,800	7	4	4	3
2,000	8	4	5	3

My target weight loss for this week is: _____.

My target weight loss for this month is: _____.

My target for protein portions per day is: _____.

I plan to add _____ additional tablespoons of pure protein powder to my shakes.

My target for fruit portions per day is: _____.

My target for vegetable portions per day is: _____.

My target for grain portions per day is: _____.

DAILY DIARY

	Shakes (2 per day)	Pure Protein Powder (TBSP)	High Protein Snack	Protein Units	Fruits	Vegetables	Grains	Water (4–6 glasses per day)
Meal 1	☐	☐☐☐		☐☐	☐☐	☐☐☐☐	☐☐	☐☐
Meal 2	☐	☐☐☐		☐☐	☐☐	☐☐☐☐	☐☐	☐☐
Meal 3	☐	☐☐☐		☐☐	☐☐	☐☐☐☐	☐☐	☐☐
Snack 1			☐	☐☐	☐☐	☐☐☐☐		☐☐
Snack 2			☐	☐☐	☐☐	☐☐☐☐		☐☐

WEEKLY DIARY

(Put a check in each box if you met your goal for the day)

	Exercise	Target Calories	Target Protein	Colorful Foods	Water
Day 1					
Day 2					
Day 3					
Day 4					
Day 5					
Day 6					
Day 7					

Suggested Reading

American Heart Association. *Fitting in Fitness: Hundreds of Simple Ways to Put More Physical Activity into Your Life.* New York: Times Books, 1997.

Brownell, K.D. *Food Fight: The Inside Story of the Food Industry, America's Obesity Crisis and What We Can Do About It.* New York: McGraw Hill, 2004.

Critser, G. *Fat Land: How Americans Became the Fattest People in the World.* Boston: Houghton Mifflin, 2003.

Eckel, R.H. *Obesity: Mechanisms and Clinical Management.* Philadelphia: Lippincott Williams & Wilkins, 2003.

Engel, C. *Wild Health: How Animals Keep Themselves Well and What We Can Learn from Them.* New York: Houghton Mifflin, 2002.

Friedman, M., and R.H. Rosenman. *Type A Behavior and Your Heart.* New York: Ballantine Books, 1974.

Nestle, M. *Food Politics: How the Food Industry Influences Nutrition and Health.* Berkeley and Los Angeles: University of California Press, 2002.

Ornish, D. *Love and Survival: The Scientific Basis for the Healing Power of Intimacy.* New York: HarperCollins, 1998.

Packer, L., M., Hiramatsu and T. Yoshikawa. *Antioxidant Food Supplements in Human Health.* San Diego: Academic Press, 1999.

Peeke, P. *Fight Fat After Forty: The Revolutionary Three-Pronged Approach That Will Break Your Stress-Fat Cycle and Make You Healthy, Fit, and Trim for Life.* New York: Viking Penguin, 2000.

Schlosser, Eric. *Fast Food Nation: The Dark Side of the All-American Meal.* New York: HarperCollins, 2002.

Willett, W.C. *Eat, Drink, and Be Healthy: The Harvard Medical School Guide to Healthy Eating.* New York: Simon and Schuster, 2001.

Acknowledgments

I would like to thank my wife, Anita, for standing by me through my entire career and the long journey of over thirty years that resulted in our wonderful children, Marc and Adrianna, and a fulfilling career and family life. I count myself among the blessed on this earth.

Susan Bowerman, my co-author, helped me not only with the recipes and menus in this book, but with lively discussions and debates on how to merge the science of nutrition and medicine with effective messages that will ring true for the reader. This is truly an M.D.-R.D. partnership. I would also like to thank my colleagues and associates at the UCLA Center for Human Nutrition, including the faculty, research fellows, and laboratory staff of the center. I also want to thank my colleagues at other universities, including Dr. Dean Ornish at the University of California, San Francisco; Dr. Pamela Peeke at the University of Maryland; Dr. James Anderson at the University of Kentucky; Dr. Herwig Ditschuneit at the University of Ulm in Germany; Dr. David Jenkins at the University of Toronto; and Dr. George Blackburn of the Harvard Medical School, for their valuable counsel and feedback on the ideas in this book.

I would like to thank the staff of the UCLA Risk Factor Obesity Clinic, especially Joe Walker and Susie Kramer, who care for hundreds of overweight patients with great compassion, and my faculty, Dr. Zhaoping Li, Mary Hardy, Susanne Henning, Diane Harris, Bill Go, Audra Lembertas, Qing-Yi Lu, and Navindra Seeram, who make it possible for our research work to create new knowledge in nutrition science.

I would also like to thank my supporters, who have made my work at the Center for Human Nutrition possible through generous donations to the Center, including Michael Milken, Lowell Milken, S. Daniel Abraham, Dr. Eddie Steinberg, Dennis Tito, Ray Stark, Lynda and Stewart Resnick, Dr. Scott Connelly, Henry Burdick, and Jane and Terry Semel. I wish to acknowledge Peter Castleman, Jim Fordyce, Michael Johnson, Greg Probert, Matt Wisk, Dr. Janice Thompson, Leslie Stanford, Dr. Jamie McManus, Audrey Sommerfeld, Rob Levy, and Jonathan Liss for embracing my philosophy and science at Herbalife International and enabling my message to go out to millions worldwide.

I would like to thank my editor at ReganBooks, Cassie Jones, who worked with me under great time pressure to be sure that the messages in this book were clear. Finally, I want to thank my publisher, the amazing Judith Regan, who believed in me and continues to inspire me with her strength, vision, and accomplishments.

Index

Index

Index

3 3 1

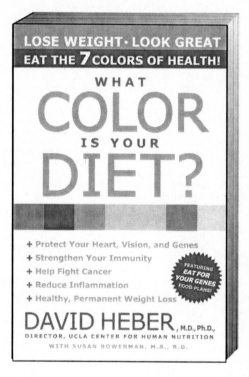

CPSIA information can be obtained at www.ICGtesting.com
Printed in the USA
LVOW08s0928220916

505673LV00008B/80/P